ACUTE & CHRONIC PANCREATITIS DIET COOKBOOK

FOR BEGINNERS

Delicious and Nutritious Recipes to Support Your Pancreatic Health and Ease Your Recovery

Kingsley Klopp

To show our appreciation for your purchase, we're delighted to offer you these special bonuses as a heartfelt thank you.

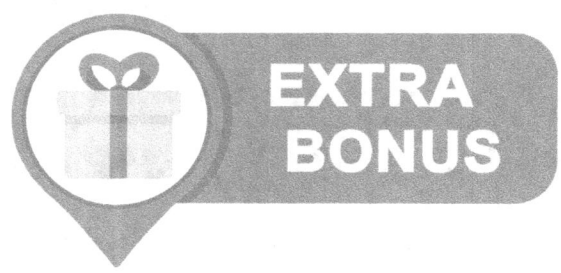

1. A Food Tracker Journal
2. Downloadable E-BOOK featuring full-color images of finished recipes

Copyright © 2024 All rights reserved.

No part of this book may be reproduced or transmitted in any form or by any means, electronic or mechanical, including photocopying, recording, or by any information storage and retrieval system, without written permission from the author. The scanning, uploading, and distribution of this book via the internet or via any other means without the permission of the author is illegal and punishable by law. The author has made every effort to ensure the accuracy of the information contained in this book. However, the author cannot be held responsible for any errors or omissions.

Table of Contents

Introduction...7

Chapter 1: Basics of Pancreatitis
- What is Acute Pancreatitis?..9
- What is Chronic Pancreatitis?..11
- Symptoms and Diagnosis...13
- Treatment Options...15

Chapter 2: Nutritional Guidelines for Pancreatitis
- Role of Nutrition in Pancreatitis Management..................18
- Foods to Avoid...21
- Foods to Include..24
- Grocery Shopping Tips..27

Breakfast Recipes
Banana Oatmeal Smoothie..31
Ginger Pear Smoothie..32
Creamy Apple-Cinnamon Smoothie.......................................33
Scrambled Egg Whites with Spinach......................................34
Zucchini and Bell Pepper Frittata..35
Apple Sauce Pancakes..36
Baked Sweet Potato Hash...37
Peach Rice Pudding..38
Savory Oatmeal with Poached Egg..39
Pumpkin Spice Oatmeal..40
Herbal Tea with Rice Cakes..41
Almond Milk Porridge..42
Buckwheat Pancakes..43
Steamed Vegetable Medley...44
Pearled Barley Porridge..45
Banana Rice Porridge...46
Egg White Omelet with Mushrooms......................................47
Quinoa and Berry Salad..48
Sweet Potato and Kale Smoothie..49

Carrot and Zucchini Muffins..50
Squash and Apple Bake..51
Warm Barley and Pumpkin Salad...52
Tapioca Pudding...53

Fish & Seafood Recipes
Poached Cod with Parsley and Lemon...54
Steamed Clams in White Wine...55
Grilled Tilapia with Herbs...56
Baked Sole with Dill..57
Shrimp and Cucumber Salad..58
Seared Scallops with Lemon Zest...59
Broiled Haddock with Rosemary...60
Herb Marinated Grilled Shrimp...61
Ginger Soy Glazed Salmon..62
Poached Trout with Mint...63
Mussels Steamed in Tomato Broth...64
Lemon Garlic Tilapia...65
Orange-Rosemary Seared Salmon..66
Prawn Stir Fry with Bell Peppers...67
Flounder with Tomato Basil Sauce...68
Seafood Paella with Brown Rice..69
Asian-Style Steamed Fish...70
Cajun Seasoned Grilled Trout...71
Clam Chowder with Skim Milk...72
Basil Lime Scallops..73
Turmeric-Ginger Marinated Halibut...74
Fish Veracruz with Tomatoes and Olives..75
Sesame Ginger Tuna Steaks..76
Steamed Blue Crabs..77
Paprika-Dusted Salmon..78

Poultry Recipes
Turkey and Mushroom Pilaf..79
Balsamic Glazed Chicken Breasts..80
Lime and Cilantro Turkey Patties..81
Salsa Fresca Chicken Bake..82
Chicken Ratatouille..83
Herb Roasted Turkey Thighs...84
Chicken Piccata without Capers..85
Grilled Turkey Breast with Cranberry Glaze..86
Chicken Cacciatore with Mushrooms...87

Orange Rosemary Chicken..88
Turkey Taco Soup...89
Chicken and Asparagus Stir Fry..90
Chicken and Broccoli Alfredo..91
Baked Turkey Cutlets with Sage...92
Chicken Soup with Barley..93
Lemon Garlic Roast Turkey...94
Turkey Spinach Meatloaf...95
Chicken and Vegetable Kebabs..96
Turkey and Quinoa Stuffed Tomatoes...97
Asian Chicken Lettuce Cups...98
Chicken Veggie Stir Fry...99
Baked Chicken with Rosemary and Thyme..100
Grilled Chicken Caesar Salad...101
Chicken and Sweet Corn Soup..102
Roasted Chicken with Apples and Onions...103
Steamed Chicken with Ginger and Scallions...104
Grilled Chicken with Herb Marinade..105

Soup & Stew Recipes
Lemon and Dill White Fish Stew...106
Garbanzo Bean and Vegetable Soup..107
Jerusalem Artichoke Soup..108
Artichoke and Potato Stew...109
Corn and Zucchini Chowder..110
Black Bean Soup with Cilantro...111
Watercress and Pea Soup...112
Beet and Cabbage Borscht..113
Green Bean and Potato Soup..114
Cauliflower and Chickpea Soup...115
Turnip and Parsnip Soup..116
Mushroom and Barley Soup...117
Fennel and Bean Stew..118
Eggplant and Tomato Stew..119
Broccoli and Lentil Soup...120
Chickpea and Spinach Soup..121
Asparagus and White Bean Soup..122
Quinoa and Vegetable Soup..123
Bean and Swiss Chard Stew..124
Red Lentil and Carrot Stew..125
Sweet Potato and Lentil Soup..126
Kale and White Bean Soup..127

Pumpkin and Bean Soup..128
Chicken and Chickpea Stew..129

10-WEEK MEAL PLAN..130

Important Note

We understand that every individual's journey with pancreatitis is unique, and the way each person responds to certain foods can vary greatly. That's why we encourage you to use this cookbook as a flexible guide. While these recipes are created to be pancreas-friendly, it's essential to personalize your meals to fit your specific nutritional needs and restrictions. Listen to your body, and don't hesitate to tweak the ingredients to suit your personal health requirements better.

As you embark on this culinary journey, remember that collaboration with your healthcare provider is key. If you ever find yourself unsure about which dietary choices are best for you, or if a particular ingredient seems to disagree with your system, consulting with your doctor or a dietitian is a wise step. They can offer guidance that is tailored specifically to your condition and help you navigate your diet safely and effectively.

Additionally, please note that the nutritional information provided alongside our recipes is approximate. Variations in ingredient choices and portion sizes can affect these values. As such, consider this information as a helpful guideline rather than an exact science, and adjust your portions and ingredients as needed to meet your specific nutritional goals.

Furthermore, If our cookbook has brought joy to your kitchen and table, we'd be thrilled to hear about your experiences in an Amazon review. On the flip side, if you stumble upon any hiccups while exploring our recipes, don't hesitate to get in touch at **kloppkingsley@gmail.com.** We're here to support your cooking journey every step of the way.

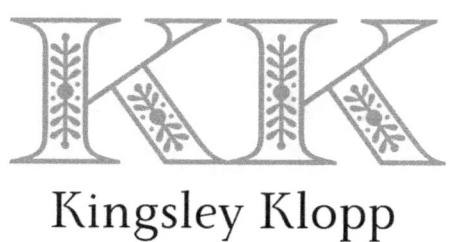

Introduction.

Welcome to your new beginning! If you, or someone you care about, is navigating the challenging waters of acute or chronic pancreatitis, this cookbook is your companion on a journey toward better health and increased comfort. You might be feeling overwhelmed or anxious about how to manage your diet, but fear not! You've just picked up a guide that will walk you through each step with ease and encouragement. Let's start with a simple truth: food is more than just sustenance. It's comfort, it's joy, and yes, it can also be medicine. When dealing with conditions like pancreatitis, understanding what to eat can transform a path filled with pain into one of recovery and wellness. This is not just a cookbook; it's a lifeline to help you harness the healing power of nutrition. Maybe you're asking yourself, "Why do I need a specialized diet?" Pancreatitis, whether acute or chronic, can significantly affect how your body handles food. This condition inflames your pancreas, which plays a crucial role in digestion and managing blood sugar. The wrong foods can aggravate symptoms, leading to discomfort and potentially serious health complications. But the right foods? They can soothe, heal, and restore. Navigating a pancreatitis-friendly diet can seem daunting. The internet is full of conflicting advice, and generic diet plans don't take into account the nuances of your condition. That's where this book comes in. We've done the heavy lifting to compile a collection of recipes that are safe, nutritious, and, most importantly, delicious. These meals are designed to support your pancreas, reduce inflammation, and make mealtime a pleasure again.

Our journey together will include everything from understanding the basics of pancreatitis and its dietary impacts to mastering flavorful dishes that support your health. We'll explore how to create balanced meals that cater to your nutritional needs without sacrificing flavor. From soothing broths and smoothies to hearty, comforting mains, every recipe is crafted to be easy on your pancreas and easy to prepare. And it's not just about avoiding pain and flare-ups. It's about finding joy in food again. Many fear that a medical diet means the end of delicious eating, but I'm here to prove that wrong. Imagine enjoying a creamy smoothie or a savory stew that not only tastes fantastic but also aligns perfectly with your health needs. That's what we aim to provide. In addition to recipes, you'll find practical tips for meal planning and grocery shopping, making it easier to maintain your diet every day. We understand that life is busy and that changes, especially dietary ones, can be hard to manage. This cookbook is designed to fit into your life, not overhaul it completely.

So, whether you're facing the diagnosis yourself or supporting a loved one, let this "Acute & Chronic Pancreatitis Diet Cookbook for Beginners" be your guide and your comfort. It's more than recipes—it's a new way to look at your diet and your health, with hope and flavor at the heart of every page.

Together, let's take the first step towards a healthier tomorrow, filled with the foods that heal. You're not alone on this journey, and with each recipe, you'll gain confidence in managing pancreatitis and reclaiming the joy of eating. Here's to a healthier, happier you!

Chapter 1: Basics of Pancreatitis

What is Acute Pancreatitis?

Acute pancreatitis is a sudden and painful inflammation of the pancreas, an organ nestled just behind your stomach. This small, yet crucial gland plays a pivotal role in digestion and blood sugar regulation, releasing enzymes and hormones that our bodies depend on. Imagine it as a diligent worker in the kitchen of your digestive system, tirelessly preparing enzymes to break down the food you eat into nutrients your body can absorb. When acute pancreatitis strikes, it's as if this hardworking organ suddenly catches fire. The enzymes it produces, designed to activate in the small intestine, start attacking the pancreas itself. This self-digestion leads to intense inflammation and swelling, causing severe abdominal pain that can radiate to your back. The pain can be relentless, a sharp reminder of how delicate and vital our internal systems are. It's not just pain that signals acute pancreatitis; it's a full-body alarm. Nausea and vomiting often accompany the discomfort, making it hard to keep anything down. Fever and a rapid pulse may follow, as your body struggles to cope with the inflammation. These symptoms can come on rapidly, sometimes within hours of a triggering event like a heavy meal or binge drinking session.

Speaking of triggers, acute pancreatitis has several common culprits. Gallstones, those tiny, hardened deposits in the gallbladder, can block the ducts leading from the pancreas, creating a pressure cooker scenario. Heavy alcohol use is another major factor, capable of damaging the pancreas over time until one day it suddenly rebels. Infections, certain medications, and even trauma to the abdomen can also provoke this painful condition. The onset of acute pancreatitis is a medical emergency. Imagine waking up in the dead of night with excruciating pain, unsure of what's happening inside your own body. The pain and uncertainty can be overwhelming. This is not something you can wait out; it's a condition that demands immediate medical attention. If left untreated, it can lead to serious complications like infected pancreatic necrosis, where parts of the pancreas die off, or systemic issues like organ failure. Treatment for acute pancreatitis typically involves hospitalization, where doctors can monitor you closely. They'll likely start by managing your pain and ensuring you stay hydrated, often through intravenous (IV) fluids. In some cases, they may need to perform procedures to remove gallstones or drain fluid collections. The goal is to give your pancreas the rest it needs to heal and to prevent any further attacks.

The emotional toll of acute pancreatitis is significant, too. It's not just the physical pain; it's the fear and anxiety of not knowing how long recovery will take, or if it might happen again. For some, this experience is a wake-up call to make lifestyle changes, such as reducing alcohol intake or adjusting their diet. For others, it's a stark reminder of how fragile our health can be, and how important it is to listen to our bodies.

Living with the memory of an acute pancreatitis attack can be daunting. Every twinge of abdominal pain might bring back the fear of a recurrence. But with proper medical care, lifestyle adjustments, and support, many people can manage their condition and lead healthy lives. Understanding the gravity of acute pancreatitis, recognizing its symptoms, and seeking prompt treatment are crucial steps in navigating this challenging health crisis.

What is Chronic Pancreatitis?

Chronic pancreatitis is a long-standing, progressive inflammation of the pancreas that gradually erodes the organ's ability to function properly. Unlike acute pancreatitis, which strikes suddenly and severely, chronic pancreatitis is a persistent condition that develops over time, often silently wreaking havoc on your digestive system and overall health. Imagine your pancreas as a diligent, lifelong worker in your body's kitchen. It produces enzymes that aid in digestion and hormones like insulin that regulate blood sugar levels. But with chronic pancreatitis, this hardworking organ faces continuous attacks, leading to scarring and irreversible damage. Over time, the pancreas becomes less effective at performing its essential tasks, and this gradual decline can feel like an ongoing battle within your body. The pain of chronic pancreatitis can be excruciating and relentless. It often starts in the upper abdomen and can radiate to your back, creating a deep, gnawing sensation that disrupts your daily life. Unlike the sudden, sharp pain of acute pancreatitis, this pain can be constant or intermittent, but it never truly goes away. It's like carrying a heavy burden that you can't set down, impacting your ability to eat, sleep, and enjoy life.

Chronic pancreatitis can lead to a myriad of symptoms beyond pain. Digestive problems are common, as the damaged pancreas struggles to produce enough enzymes to break down food. This can cause malabsorption, leading to weight loss, diarrhea, and fatty stools. The lack of proper digestion means your body isn't getting the nutrients it needs, leaving you feeling weak and fatigued. Diabetes is another serious complication of chronic pancreatitis. As the disease progresses, the insulin-producing cells in the pancreas are destroyed, leading to high blood sugar levels. Managing both chronic pancreatitis and diabetes can be incredibly challenging, requiring careful monitoring of diet and medication. The causes of chronic pancreatitis are varied, with alcohol abuse being one of the most common. Long-term heavy drinking can poison the pancreas, leading to inflammation and scarring. Genetic factors also play a role, and some people inherit conditions that predispose them to chronic pancreatitis. Autoimmune diseases, where the body's immune system attacks its own tissues, can also cause this persistent inflammation.

Living with chronic pancreatitis is an emotional and physical rollercoaster. The uncertainty of flare-ups, the constant pain, and the fear of complications weigh heavily on those affected. It's a daily struggle that affects not just the individual but their loved ones as well. Relationships can be strained as the illness takes its toll, and the emotional burden can lead to feelings of isolation and depression.

Treatment for chronic pancreatitis focuses on managing pain, improving digestion, and addressing complications like diabetes. Pain management can include medications, nerve blocks, and sometimes surgery to remove part of the pancreas or relieve pressure on the ducts. Enzyme replacement therapy helps with digestion, allowing your body to absorb nutrients more effectively. Dietary changes are crucial, with a focus on low-fat meals and avoiding alcohol entirely. Support is vital for those living with chronic pancreatitis. Connecting with others who understand your experience can provide emotional relief and practical advice. Support groups, both in-person and online, offer a sense of community and understanding that is invaluable. It's important to remember that while chronic pancreatitis is a serious and life-altering condition, there is hope. Advances in medical treatment and a deeper understanding of the disease mean that better management strategies are available. By working closely with healthcare providers, making necessary lifestyle changes, and seeking support, individuals with chronic pancreatitis can improve their quality of life.

Facing chronic pancreatitis is undeniably tough, but resilience and determination can make a significant difference. It's about finding the strength to adapt, seeking out the resources and support you need, and holding onto hope even in the darkest moments. You are more than your illness, and with the right care and support, you can navigate this challenging journey and find moments of peace and joy amidst the struggle.

Symptoms and Diagnosis

Pancreatitis, whether acute or chronic, presents a challenging medical condition marked by inflammation of the pancreas. The symptoms and diagnostic approaches for each type differ significantly, reflecting the distinct nature and progression of these diseases.

Symptoms of Acute Pancreatitis

Acute pancreatitis is characterized by a sudden onset of symptoms, often following a heavy meal or binge drinking. The hallmark symptom is severe abdominal pain, typically located in the upper abdomen and radiating to the back. This pain can be intense, constant, and debilitating, often requiring emergency medical attention.

Other symptoms include:

- Nausea and Vomiting: Accompanying the abdominal pain, these symptoms can make it difficult to keep food or liquids down, exacerbating dehydration.
- Fever: A mild to moderate fever is common as the body responds to the inflammation.
- Rapid Pulse: An elevated heart rate often indicates the body's distress.
- Tenderness and Swelling: The abdomen may be tender to the touch and visibly swollen.
- Jaundice: If a gallstone blocks the bile duct, jaundice (yellowing of the skin and eyes) may occur.

The intensity and combination of these symptoms can vary, but the sudden, severe abdominal pain is a consistent and alarming feature that should prompt immediate medical evaluation.

Symptoms of Chronic Pancreatitis

Chronic pancreatitis develops gradually and is characterized by persistent inflammation leading to permanent damage to the pancreas. The symptoms can be more subtle and protracted compared to acute pancreatitis but are equally disruptive to a person's life.

Key symptoms include:

- Chronic Abdominal Pain: Unlike the sudden onset in acute pancreatitis, the pain in chronic pancreatitis is more continuous, often described as a dull ache that may become more intense after eating. This pain can radiate to the back and is a constant reminder of the underlying condition.
- Digestive Issues: As the pancreas becomes less effective at producing digestive enzymes, symptoms like diarrhea, greasy or fatty stools (steatorrhea), and weight loss become prevalent. The body struggles to absorb nutrients, leading to malnutrition.
- Diabetes: Chronic pancreatitis can impair insulin production, resulting in diabetes. Symptoms of diabetes such as increased thirst, frequent urination, and unexplained weight loss may develop.

- Fatigue and Weakness: The chronic pain and malnutrition associated with pancreatitis can lead to persistent fatigue and a general feeling of weakness.

Diagnosis of Acute Pancreatitis

Diagnosing acute pancreatitis requires a combination of medical history, physical examination, and diagnostic tests:
- **Medical History and Physical Examination:** Doctors will ask about the onset and nature of symptoms, recent alcohol consumption, and any history of gallstones. A physical examination will focus on abdominal tenderness and signs of jaundice.
- **Blood Tests:** Elevated levels of pancreatic enzymes (amylase and lipase) in the blood are a key indicator of acute pancreatitis. Other blood tests can reveal signs of inflammation, dehydration, and organ function.
- **Imaging Tests:**
  - Ultrasound: Often the first imaging test, it can detect gallstones and other abnormalities.
  - CT Scan: Provides detailed images of the pancreas and surrounding structures, helping to confirm the diagnosis and assess the extent of inflammation.
  - MRI: Sometimes used to get a more detailed view of the pancreas and ducts.

Diagnosis of Chronic Pancreatitis

The diagnosis of chronic pancreatitis involves more extensive investigation due to its gradual onset and the complexity of symptoms:
- **Medical History and Physical Examination:** Chronic pancreatitis requires a detailed medical history focusing on alcohol consumption, family history, and the pattern of symptoms. A physical exam will assess nutritional status and abdominal tenderness.
- **Blood Tests:** Unlike acute pancreatitis, enzyme levels in chronic pancreatitis may be normal. Blood tests focus on indicators of malnutrition, liver function, and blood sugar levels.
- **Stool Tests:** To assess fat malabsorption, stool tests can measure the amount of fat present, which is a sign of insufficient digestive enzymes.
- **Imaging Tests:**
  - CT Scan or MRI: These imaging tests help visualize calcifications in the pancreas, ductal abnormalities, and other structural changes.
  - Endoscopic Ultrasound (EUS): An advanced procedure providing detailed images of the pancreas and surrounding tissues.
  - MRCP (Magnetic Resonance Cholangiopancreatography): A specialized MRI technique to visualize the pancreatic and bile ducts.

Treatment Options

Treating pancreatitis, whether acute or chronic, requires a multifaceted approach that addresses the inflammation, manages pain, and aims to prevent complications. The treatment strategies differ based on the severity and nature of the condition, but the ultimate goal is to restore pancreatic function and improve the patient's quality of life.

Treatment for Acute Pancreatitis

Acute pancreatitis typically requires hospitalization due to the sudden and severe nature of the condition. The primary objectives during treatment are to stabilize the patient, manage pain, and prevent complications.

1. **Hospitalization and Initial Care:**
   - Fasting: Patients are often advised to fast initially to rest the pancreas. This means no food or drink, allowing the pancreas to recover without being stimulated to produce enzymes.
   - IV Fluids: To prevent dehydration and maintain blood pressure, patients receive intravenous (IV) fluids.
   - Pain Management: Pain relief is a crucial aspect of treatment. Medications such as acetaminophen, NSAIDs, or opioids may be used, depending on the severity of the pain.

2. **Nutritional Support:**
   - Gradual Reintroduction of Food: Once the inflammation subsides, a gradual reintroduction of food begins, starting with clear liquids and progressing to solid foods.
   - Enteral Nutrition: In severe cases where fasting is prolonged, a feeding tube may be used to deliver nutrients directly to the small intestine, bypassing the pancreas.

3. **Treating Underlying Causes:**
   - Gallstones: If gallstones are the cause, procedures such as endoscopic retrograde cholangiopancreatography (ERCP) can remove the stones. In some cases, surgery to remove the gallbladder (cholecystectomy) is necessary.
   - Alcohol Consumption: For alcohol-induced pancreatitis, complete abstinence from alcohol is critical.

4. **Monitoring and Managing Complications:**
   - Infections: If pancreatic tissue becomes infected, antibiotics are administered, and in some cases, surgical drainage or debridement may be required.
   - Systemic Complications: Acute pancreatitis can lead to complications like respiratory failure, kidney failure, or cardiovascular issues, which require intensive care and supportive treatment.

Treatment for Chronic Pancreatitis

Chronic pancreatitis requires a long-term management plan that focuses on controlling symptoms, managing complications, and maintaining nutritional health.

1. Pain Management:
- Medications: Non-opioid pain relievers are preferred initially. Opioids may be used for severe pain, but long-term use is avoided due to the risk of dependency.
- Nerve Blocks: For persistent pain, procedures such as celiac plexus block can provide relief by blocking pain signals from the pancreas.
- Surgical Interventions: In some cases, surgical procedures like the Puestow procedure (pancreaticojejunostomy) can help by creating a drainage route for pancreatic enzymes, relieving pressure and pain.

2. Enzyme Replacement Therapy:
- Pancreatic Enzymes: Oral enzyme supplements are prescribed to aid digestion and improve nutrient absorption, addressing malnutrition and digestive symptoms.

3. Nutritional Support:
- Dietary Changes: A low-fat diet is recommended to reduce pancreatic stimulation. Patients are advised to eat small, frequent meals to minimize digestive strain.
- Vitamin and Mineral Supplements: Due to malabsorption, supplements may be necessary to address deficiencies in fat-soluble vitamins (A, D, E, K) and minerals like calcium and magnesium.

4. Managing Diabetes:
- Insulin Therapy: As chronic pancreatitis can lead to diabetes, patients may require insulin to manage blood sugar levels.
- Blood Sugar Monitoring: Regular monitoring and adjusting dietary intake are essential for managing diabetes secondary to pancreatitis.

5. Addressing Underlying Causes:
- Alcohol Abstinence: Complete avoidance of alcohol is crucial for preventing further pancreatic damage.
- Lifestyle Modifications: Smoking cessation and maintaining a healthy weight are recommended to reduce the risk of exacerbations.

6. Treating Complications:
- Pancreatic Pseudocysts: These fluid-filled sacs can develop in the pancreas. Treatment options include drainage, either endoscopically or surgically.
- Biliary Obstruction: If the bile duct is blocked, procedures like ERCP or surgical bypass may be needed to restore bile flow.

7. Psychological and Emotional Support:
- Counseling and Support Groups: Chronic pain and the lifestyle changes required for managing chronic pancreatitis can be mentally and emotionally taxing. Psychological counseling and support groups can provide significant emotional support and coping strategies.

8. Monitoring and Follow-Up:
- Regular Medical Check-Ups: Ongoing monitoring is essential to manage chronic pancreatitis effectively. Regular check-ups help track the progression of the disease, adjust treatments, and detect complications early.

Hence, the treatment of acute and chronic pancreatitis is a complex and dynamic process, requiring a tailored approach based on the severity and progression of the disease. For acute pancreatitis, immediate medical intervention is crucial to stabilize the patient and address the underlying causes. In contrast, chronic pancreatitis demands a long-term, comprehensive management plan that includes pain control, nutritional support, enzyme replacement, and lifestyle modifications.

Chapter 2: Nutritional Guidelines for Pancreatitis

Role of Nutrition in Pancreatitis Management

Nutrition plays a pivotal role in managing pancreatitis, a condition marked by inflammation of the pancreas. The journey through pancreatitis can be arduous and emotionally taxing, and understanding the importance of nutrition can empower individuals to take control of their health and improve their quality of life. Whether dealing with the sudden onset of acute pancreatitis or the long-term challenges of chronic pancreatitis, proper nutrition is a cornerstone of effective management and recovery.

The Emotional Impact of Dietary Changes

When diagnosed with pancreatitis, the prospect of changing your diet can feel overwhelming. Food is not just fuel; it's a source of comfort, joy, and social connection. Adapting to a new way of eating requires not only physical adjustments but also emotional resilience. However, embracing these changes can significantly alleviate symptoms, prevent complications, and foster a sense of empowerment and control over your health journey.

Nutritional Needs in Acute Pancreatitis

In the case of acute pancreatitis, the pancreas needs time to rest and recover from the inflammation. This often means abstaining from food and drink initially, which can be a difficult and distressing experience. The following nutritional strategies are essential during the acute phase:

1. Fasting and IV Fluids:
- Initial Fasting: The first step is usually complete fasting to reduce pancreatic stimulation. This allows the pancreas to heal without the burden of digesting food.
- Intravenous (IV) Fluids: To prevent dehydration and maintain electrolyte balance, patients receive fluids through an IV. This support is vital for stabilizing the body during the initial acute phase.

2. Gradual Reintroduction of Food:
- Clear Liquids: Once inflammation subsides, clear liquids like broth, gelatin, and water are introduced. This step is taken cautiously to ensure the pancreas can handle small amounts of food without becoming irritated.
- Soft, Low-Fat Foods: Gradually, soft and low-fat foods are reintroduced, such as applesauce, rice, and boiled vegetables. This helps ease the pancreas back into its digestive role without overstressing it.

Nutritional Management in Chronic Pancreatitis

Chronic pancreatitis requires a long-term dietary strategy that supports pancreatic function, manages symptoms, and prevents malnutrition. The following guidelines are crucial for those living with chronic pancreatitis:

1. Low-Fat Diet:
- Reducing Fat Intake: A diet low in fat is essential to minimize the workload on the pancreas. Fatty foods can trigger pancreatic enzyme production, leading to pain and inflammation.
- Healthy Alternatives: Incorporating healthy fats from sources like avocados, nuts, and olive oil in moderation can provide necessary nutrients without overwhelming the pancreas.

2. Small, Frequent Meals:
- Easing Digestion: Eating small, frequent meals helps manage symptoms by preventing the pancreas from becoming overstimulated. This approach can also help maintain steady blood sugar levels and energy throughout the day.
- Balanced Nutrition: Ensuring each meal is balanced with carbohydrates, proteins, and a small amount of healthy fats supports overall health and prevents nutritional deficiencies.

3. Enzyme Replacement Therapy:
- Digestive Enzymes: For those with chronic pancreatitis, the pancreas may not produce enough enzymes to digest food properly. Pancreatic enzyme supplements can help improve digestion and nutrient absorption, alleviating symptoms like diarrhea and weight loss.

4. Vitamin and Mineral Supplements:
- Addressing Deficiencies: Malabsorption can lead to deficiencies in essential vitamins and minerals, particularly fat-soluble vitamins (A, D, E, K). Supplements can help correct these deficiencies and prevent complications like osteoporosis.
- Personalized Supplement Plans: Working with a healthcare provider to develop a tailored supplement plan ensures that individual nutritional needs are met.

Emotional and Psychological Support

The emotional toll of pancreatitis and the necessary dietary changes cannot be underestimated. It's essential to address the psychological aspects of managing this condition:

1. Emotional Resilience:
- Acceptance and Adaptation: Accepting the need for dietary changes and adapting to a new way of eating can be emotionally challenging. Finding healthy, enjoyable foods that fit within dietary guidelines can make this transition easier.
- Mindful Eating: Practicing mindful eating, where you focus on the taste, texture, and enjoyment of each bite, can help create a positive relationship with food despite the restrictions.

2. **Social Support:**
- Family and Friends: Engaging family and friends in your dietary journey can provide emotional support and make social situations easier to navigate. Sharing meals that fit your dietary needs can help maintain social connections and reduce feelings of isolation.
- Support Groups: Joining support groups, either in person or online, can connect you with others who understand the challenges of living with pancreatitis. Sharing experiences, tips, and encouragement can be incredibly beneficial.

In summary, nutrition is a fundamental aspect of managing pancreatitis, influencing both physical health and emotional well-being. While the dietary changes required can be daunting, they are crucial for reducing symptoms, preventing complications, and improving quality of life. By embracing a low-fat diet, incorporating small, frequent meals, and utilizing enzyme and vitamin supplements, individuals can support their pancreatic health and take control of their condition.

Foods to Avoid

Managing pancreatitis, whether acute or chronic, involves making significant dietary changes to reduce inflammation and prevent further damage to the pancreas. Understanding which foods to avoid is crucial for controlling symptoms, promoting healing, and maintaining overall health. Adapting to these dietary restrictions can be challenging, but it's a vital step towards managing the condition effectively and improving quality of life.

The Importance of Avoiding Certain Foods
When the pancreas is inflamed, it needs time to heal and rest. Consuming foods that are difficult to digest or that stimulate the pancreas to produce digestive enzymes can exacerbate symptoms and lead to complications. Therefore, avoiding specific foods is essential to reduce the workload on the pancreas and to prevent pain and further inflammation.

High-Fat Foods
High-fat foods are particularly problematic for individuals with pancreatitis. Fatty foods stimulate the pancreas to release digestive enzymes, which can increase inflammation and pain.

1. Fried and Greasy Foods:
- Examples: French fries, fried chicken, doughnuts, and other deep-fried items.
- Impact: These foods are difficult to digest and can trigger pancreatic enzyme secretion, leading to increased pain and inflammation.

2. High-Fat Meats:
- Examples: Bacon, sausage, fatty cuts of beef or pork, and processed meats like salami.
- Impact: These meats contain high levels of saturated fat, which can strain the pancreas and worsen symptoms.

3. Full-Fat Dairy Products:
- Examples: Whole milk, cream, butter, full-fat cheese, and ice cream.
- Impact: These products are rich in fat, which can be challenging for the pancreas to process.

Sugary and Refined Carbohydrates
Sugary and refined carbohydrates can also be detrimental to those with pancreatitis. These foods can lead to spikes in blood sugar levels and can contribute to the development of diabetes, a common complication of chronic pancreatitis.

1. Sugary Snacks and Desserts:
- Examples: Candy, cookies, cakes, pastries, and sweetened beverages like soda.
- Impact: High sugar content can lead to rapid increases in blood sugar, placing additional stress on the pancreas.

2. Refined Grains:
- Examples: White bread, white rice, and pasta made from refined flour.
- Impact: These foods lack fiber and essential nutrients, leading to quick digestion and absorption, which can affect blood sugar control.

Alcohol

Alcohol is one of the most significant dietary factors to avoid for individuals with pancreatitis. It is a major cause of pancreatitis and can exacerbate existing conditions, leading to severe complications.

1. All Alcoholic Beverages:
- Examples: Beer, wine, spirits, and cocktails.
- Impact: Alcohol can cause direct damage to pancreatic cells, increase inflammation, and interfere with the pancreas's ability to function properly. Even small amounts of alcohol can trigger a pancreatitis flare-up.

Processed and Fast Foods

Processed and fast foods often contain unhealthy fats, sugars, and additives that can aggravate pancreatitis symptoms.

1. Processed Foods:
- Examples: Packaged snacks, frozen meals, and processed cheese products.
- Impact: These foods typically contain high levels of unhealthy fats, sugars, and preservatives that can increase the workload on the pancreas.

2. Fast Foods:
- Examples: Burgers, fries, pizza, and other quick-serve restaurant items.
- Impact: Fast foods are usually high in trans fats and other unhealthy ingredients that can trigger pancreatitis symptoms and contribute to inflammation.

Spicy Foods and Irritants

Spicy foods and other dietary irritants can exacerbate the symptoms of pancreatitis by irritating the digestive tract.

1. Spicy Foods:
- Examples: Hot peppers, spicy sauces, and dishes with heavy seasoning.
- Impact: These foods can cause discomfort and increase inflammation in the digestive tract.

2. Caffeinated Beverages:
- Examples: Coffee, energy drinks, and some teas.
- Impact: Caffeine can stimulate gastric acid secretion and irritate the digestive system, potentially worsening pancreatitis symptoms.

High-Fiber Foods
While fiber is generally beneficial for digestion, certain high-fiber foods can be challenging for individuals with pancreatitis, especially during flare-ups.

1. Raw Vegetables and Fruits:
- Examples: Raw broccoli, cauliflower, and apples with skin.
- Impact: These foods can be hard to digest and may cause bloating and discomfort.

2. Whole Grains:
- Examples: Brown rice, whole wheat bread, and bran.
- Impact: High-fiber grains can be tough to digest and might lead to gastrointestinal distress.

Navigating dietary restrictions with pancreatitis involves understanding and avoiding foods that can exacerbate symptoms and cause further damage to the pancreas. While it can be challenging to adapt to these changes, focusing on a diet that supports pancreatic health is crucial for managing the condition and improving overall well-being. By avoiding high-fat foods, sugary and refined carbohydrates, alcohol, processed and fast foods, spicy foods, and certain high-fiber foods, individuals with pancreatitis can reduce inflammation, alleviate pain, and support their body's healing process. It's important to work closely with healthcare providers and nutritionists to develop a tailored diet plan that meets individual needs and preferences.

Foods to Include

Managing pancreatitis through diet involves carefully selecting foods that are easy on the pancreas while providing essential nutrients for overall health. The right foods can help reduce inflammation, manage symptoms, and promote healing. Embracing these dietary changes can be challenging, but they are crucial for living well with pancreatitis and improving quality of life.

Importance of a Pancreatitis-Friendly Diet

A pancreatitis-friendly diet is designed to minimize stress on the pancreas, reduce inflammation, and prevent flare-ups. This diet typically includes low-fat, nutrient-dense foods that are easy to digest. These foods provide the necessary energy and nutrients without overstimulating the pancreas, helping to manage symptoms and support recovery.

Lean Protein Sources

Protein is essential for repair and maintenance of body tissues, including the pancreas. However, it's important to choose lean sources of protein to avoid excessive fat intake.

1. Skinless Poultry:
- Examples: Chicken breast, turkey breast.
- Benefits: These are low in fat and high in protein, making them gentle on the pancreas while providing essential nutrients.

2. Fish and Seafood:
- Examples: Cod, tilapia, salmon (in moderation), shrimp.
- Benefits: Fish and seafood are excellent sources of lean protein and contain healthy omega-3 fatty acids, which can reduce inflammation.

3. Plant-Based Proteins:
- Examples: Tofu, tempeh, legumes (lentils, beans).
- Benefits: Plant-based proteins are low in fat and high in fiber, providing a nutritious alternative to animal proteins.

Low-Fat Dairy Alternatives

Dairy products can be included in a pancreatitis-friendly diet if they are low in fat. Full-fat dairy can be hard to digest and may trigger symptoms, so opting for low-fat or fat-free options is crucial.

1. Low-Fat Yogurt:
- Examples: Greek yogurt (low-fat or fat-free).
- Benefits: Provides probiotics for digestive health and is a good source of calcium and protein.

2. **Skim or Low-Fat Milk:**
   - Examples: Skim milk, 1% milk.
   - Benefits: These provide calcium and vitamin D without the high fat content of whole milk.
3. **Low-Fat Cheese:**
   - Examples: Cottage cheese, part-skim mozzarella.
   - Benefits: These cheeses offer protein and calcium with less fat.

Fruits and Vegetables

Fruits and vegetables are rich in vitamins, minerals, and antioxidants, which are essential for overall health. They are generally low in fat and calories, making them ideal for a pancreatitis-friendly diet.

1. **Non-Starchy Vegetables:**
   - Examples: Leafy greens (spinach, kale), broccoli, bell peppers, carrots.
   - Benefits: These vegetables are low in calories and high in fiber, vitamins, and minerals. They can be eaten raw, steamed, or roasted.
2. **Fruits:**
   - Examples: Berries (blueberries, strawberries), apples (without the skin), melons.
   - Benefits: Fruits provide natural sweetness, vitamins, and antioxidants. They should be consumed in moderation and preferably fresh or frozen without added sugar.

Whole Grains

Whole grains are an excellent source of fiber, which aids digestion and helps maintain stable blood sugar levels. They are also rich in vitamins and minerals.

1. **Whole Grain Breads and Cereals:**
   - Examples: Whole wheat bread, oatmeal, brown rice, quinoa.
   - Benefits: These grains provide sustained energy and important nutrients while being gentle on the digestive system.
2. **Pasta:**
   - Examples: Whole grain pasta, brown rice pasta.
   - Benefits: Whole grain pasta is a good source of fiber and can be part of a balanced diet when consumed in moderation.

Healthy Fats

While a low-fat diet is essential for managing pancreatitis, some healthy fats can be included in moderation. These fats are important for overall health and can help reduce inflammation.

1. **Avocado:**
   - Benefits: Avocados are rich in healthy monounsaturated fats and provide essential vitamins and minerals.

2. Nuts and Seeds:
- Examples: Almonds, flaxseeds, chia seeds (in small quantities).
- Benefits: These are good sources of omega-3 fatty acids and fiber. They should be consumed in moderation due to their high-fat content.

3. Olive Oil:
- Benefits: Olive oil is a healthy source of fat that can be used in cooking or as a salad dressing. It contains anti-inflammatory properties and is easy to digest.

Hydration

Staying hydrated is crucial for overall health and can help manage pancreatitis symptoms.

1. Water:
- Benefits: Drinking plenty of water helps maintain hydration and supports overall bodily functions.

2. Herbal Teas:
- Examples: Chamomile, peppermint, ginger tea.
- Benefits: Herbal teas can soothe the digestive system and provide hydration without the caffeine found in some other beverages.

Nutrient-Dense Snacks

Healthy snacks can provide additional nutrients and help maintain energy levels throughout the day.

1. Fresh Fruits and Vegetables:
- Examples: Apple slices, carrot sticks, celery with a small amount of almond butter.
- Benefits: These snacks are low in calories and high in essential nutrients.

2. Low-Fat Yogurt or Cottage Cheese:
- Benefits: These snacks provide protein and calcium, which are important for maintaining muscle mass and bone health.

3. Smoothies:
- Examples: Smoothies made with low-fat yogurt, fresh fruits, and a handful of spinach.
- Benefits: Smoothies can be a delicious way to include a variety of nutrients in your diet. They should be made with low-fat ingredients and no added sugars.

Grocery Shopping Tips

Grocery shopping can be a daunting task for individuals managing pancreatitis, as it requires careful selection of foods that are gentle on the pancreas while providing essential nutrients. With the right strategies and planning, shopping can become a more manageable and even enjoyable part of maintaining a pancreatitis-friendly diet.

Planning Ahead
Effective grocery shopping starts with planning. This ensures that you buy only what you need, which helps you avoid impulse purchases that may not be pancreatitis-friendly.

1. Create a Meal Plan:
- Weekly Planning: Plan your meals and snacks for the week. This helps you create a comprehensive shopping list and ensures you have all the ingredients needed for nutritious, pancreatitis-friendly meals.
- Variety and Balance: Ensure your meal plan includes a variety of foods to provide balanced nutrition. Include lean proteins, low-fat dairy, fruits, vegetables, whole grains, and healthy fats.

2. Make a Shopping List:
- Organize by Sections: Write your list according to the layout of the grocery store (e.g., produce, dairy, meats, grains). This makes shopping more efficient and helps you avoid missing items.
- Stick to the List: Having a list helps you stay focused and reduces the temptation to buy unhealthy or impulsive items.

Reading Labels
Reading food labels is crucial for making informed choices. Labels provide valuable information about the nutritional content of foods, helping you avoid items that can aggravate pancreatitis symptoms.

1. Check the Fat Content:
- Low-Fat Options: Look for products labeled as low-fat, fat-free, or reduced-fat. These are typically better choices for individuals with pancreatitis.
- Avoid Trans Fats: Steer clear of products containing trans fats, which are often listed as partially hydrogenated oils.

2. Monitor Sugar Levels:
- Low Sugar: Choose products with little to no added sugars. High sugar intake can exacerbate inflammation and contribute to other health issues like diabetes.
- Hidden Sugars: Be aware of hidden sugars in products like sauces, dressings, and processed foods. Ingredients ending in "-ose" (e.g., glucose, fructose) are forms of sugar.

3. Look for Fiber:
- Whole Grains: Opt for whole grain products with higher fiber content. Whole grains like brown rice, quinoa, and whole wheat bread are nutritious and support digestive health.
- Soluble Fiber: Foods rich in soluble fiber, such as oats and legumes, can help manage blood sugar levels and improve digestion.

Shopping for Lean Proteins
Lean proteins are essential for repairing and maintaining body tissues without putting excessive strain on the pancreas.

1. Poultry and Fish:
- Skinless Poultry: Choose skinless chicken or turkey breasts. These are low in fat and high in protein.
- Fish: Select lean fish like cod, tilapia, and haddock. Fatty fish like salmon can be included in moderation due to their healthy omega-3 fatty acids.

2. Plant-Based Proteins:
- Legumes: Beans, lentils, and chickpeas are excellent sources of plant-based protein and fiber.
- Tofu and Tempeh: These are versatile and nutritious alternatives to meat, providing protein without the fat content.

3. Low-Fat Dairy:
- Yogurt and Milk: Opt for low-fat or fat-free versions of yogurt and milk. Greek yogurt is a good choice for its higher protein content.
- Cheese: Choose low-fat or part-skim cheeses like mozzarella and cottage cheese.

Selecting Fruits and Vegetables
Fruits and vegetables are vital for providing vitamins, minerals, and antioxidants that support overall health and reduce inflammation.

1. Fresh Produce:
- Variety: Aim to include a variety of colors and types of fruits and vegetables in your diet. Each color represents different nutrients and antioxidants.
- Seasonal Produce: Choose seasonal fruits and vegetables for the freshest and most nutrient-rich options.

2. Frozen and Canned Options:
- Frozen Vegetables: These are often just as nutritious as fresh ones and can be convenient for quick meals. Look for options without added sauces or seasoning.
- Canned Produce: Select canned fruits packed in water or their own juice, not syrup. For vegetables, choose those without added salt.

Whole Grains and Healthy Carbs

Whole grains and healthy carbohydrates provide sustained energy and are important for a balanced diet.

1. Whole Grain Products:
   - Bread and Pasta: Choose whole grain or whole wheat bread and pasta. These contain more fiber and nutrients than refined versions.
   - Cereal and Oats: Look for whole grain cereals and oats. Avoid those with high sugar content.
2. Rice and Quinoa:
   - Brown Rice: A better option than white rice due to its higher fiber content.
   - Quinoa: A complete protein that is also rich in fiber and easy to digest.

Healthy Fats

While a low-fat diet is essential for managing pancreatitis, incorporating small amounts of healthy fats is important.

1. Avocado:
   - Nutrient-Rich: Avocados provide healthy monounsaturated fats and essential vitamins. Use them in moderation.
2. Nuts and Seeds:
   - Moderation: Include small amounts of nuts and seeds like almonds, flaxseeds, and chia seeds. They provide healthy fats and fiber but should be consumed in moderation.
3. Oils:
   - Olive Oil: Use olive oil for cooking or as a salad dressing. It is a healthy source of fat with anti-inflammatory properties.
   - Cooking Sprays: Consider using cooking sprays instead of pouring oil to better control the amount used.

Hydration and Beverages

Staying hydrated is crucial for overall health and digestive function.

1. Water:
   - Primary Beverage: Make water your main beverage choice. It helps maintain hydration and supports all bodily functions.
   - Infused Water: For variety, infuse water with slices of fruit, cucumber, or herbs for a refreshing twist.
2. Herbal Teas:
   - Caffeine-Free: Herbal teas like chamomile, peppermint, and ginger are soothing and can support digestive health.
3. Avoid Sugary Drinks:
   - Soda and Juice: Limit or avoid sugary sodas and fruit juices, which can contribute to inflammation and digestive issues.

Navigating the Grocery Store

Shopping can be more efficient and less stressful with a few simple strategies:

1. Shop the Perimeter:
   - Perimeter First: The outer aisles of the grocery store typically contain fresh produce, dairy, and meats. Start here to fill your cart with whole, nutritious foods.
   - Inner Aisles: Venture into the inner aisles for specific items like whole grains, canned goods, and frozen foods, but stick to your list to avoid processed foods.
2. Shop When You're Not Hungry:
   - Avoid Impulse Buys: Shopping on a full stomach can help you avoid impulse purchases of unhealthy snacks and convenience foods.
3. Read Labels:
   - Ingredient Lists: Choose products with simple, recognizable ingredients. Avoid those with long lists of additives, preservatives, and artificial ingredients.

Breakfast Recipes

1. Banana Oatmeal Smoothie

Ingredients:
- 1 ripe banana
- 1/2 cup rolled oats
- 1 cup unsweetened almond milk
- 1 tablespoon almond butter
- 1 teaspoon honey (optional)
- 1/2 teaspoon vanilla extract
- 1/2 teaspoon ground cinnamon
- 1/2 cup ice cubes

Instructions:
1. Place the rolled oats in a blender and pulse until finely ground.
2. Add the banana, almond milk, almond butter, honey (if using), vanilla extract, ground cinnamon, and ice cubes to the blender.
3. Blend until smooth and creamy.
4. Pour into a glass and serve immediately.

Nutrition Info (per serving):
- Calories: 300
- Protein: 7g
- Carbohydrates: 49g
- Fat: 9g
- Fiber: 6g
- Sugar: 17g

Serves: 1
Cooking Time: 5 minutes

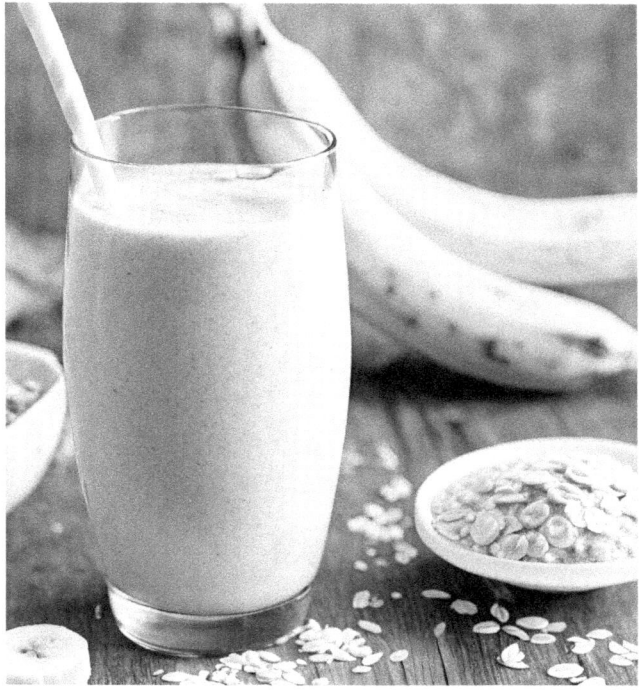

2. Ginger Pear Smoothie

Ingredients:
- 1 ripe pear, cored and chopped
- 1/2 cup plain low-fat yogurt
- 1/2 cup unsweetened almond milk
- 1 teaspoon grated fresh ginger
- 1 tablespoon honey (optional)
- 1/2 teaspoon ground cinnamon
- 1/2 cup ice cubes

Instructions:
1. Add the chopped pear, yogurt, almond milk, grated ginger, honey (if using), ground cinnamon, and ice cubes to a blender.
2. Blend until smooth and creamy.
3. Pour into a glass and serve immediately.

Nutrition Info (per serving):
- Calories: 180
- Protein: 5g
- Carbohydrates: 36g
- Fat: 3g
- Fiber: 4g
- Sugar: 26g

Serves: 1
Cooking Time: 5 minutes

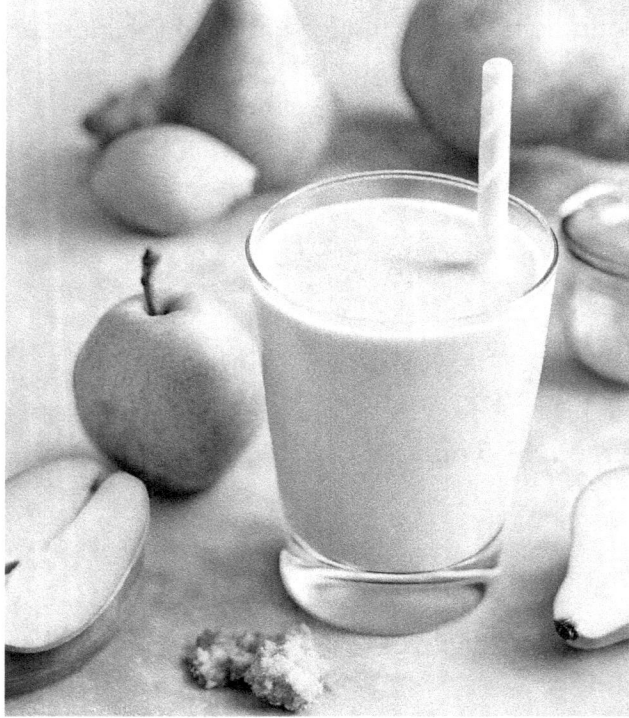

3. Creamy Apple-Cinnamon Smoothie

Ingredients:
- 1 apple, cored and chopped
- 1/2 cup plain low-fat yogurt
- 1/2 cup unsweetened almond milk
- 1 tablespoon almond butter
- 1 teaspoon honey (optional)
- 1/2 teaspoon ground cinnamon
- 1/4 teaspoon nutmeg
- 1/2 cup ice cubes

Instructions:
1. Add the chopped apple, yogurt, almond milk, almond butter, honey (if using), ground cinnamon, nutmeg, and ice cubes to a blender.
2. Blend until smooth and creamy.
3. Pour into a glass and serve immediately.

Nutrition Info (per serving):
- Calories: 210
- Protein: 6g
- Carbohydrates: 35g
- Fat: 7g
- Fiber: 4g
- Sugar: 24g

Serves: 1
Cooking Time: 5 minutes

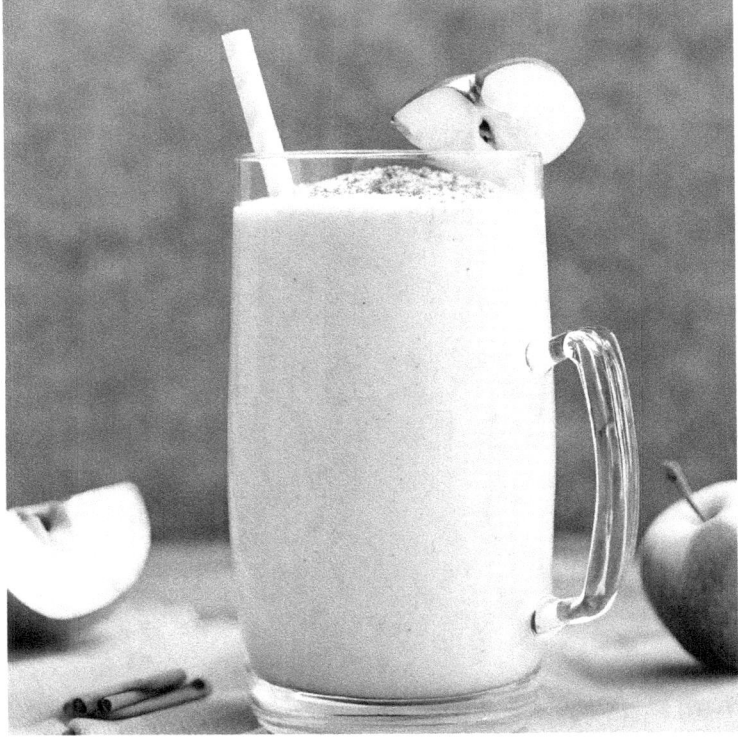

4. Scrambled Egg Whites with Spinach

Ingredients:
- 4 large egg whites
- 1 cup fresh spinach, chopped
- 1/4 cup low-fat milk
- 1 tablespoon olive oil
- 1/4 teaspoon garlic powder
- 1/4 teaspoon onion powder

Instructions:
1. In a bowl, whisk together the egg whites, low-fat milk, garlic powder, and onion powder.
2. Heat the olive oil in a non-stick skillet over medium heat.
3. Add the chopped spinach to the skillet and sauté until wilted, about 2-3 minutes.
4. Pour the egg white mixture into the skillet with the spinach.
5. Cook, stirring gently, until the egg whites are set, about 3-4 minutes.
6. Serve immediately.

Nutrition Info (per serving):
- Calories: 120
- Protein: 12g
- Carbohydrates: 4g
- Fat: 7g
- Fiber: 1g
- Sugar: 2g

Serves: 1
Cooking Time: 10 minutes

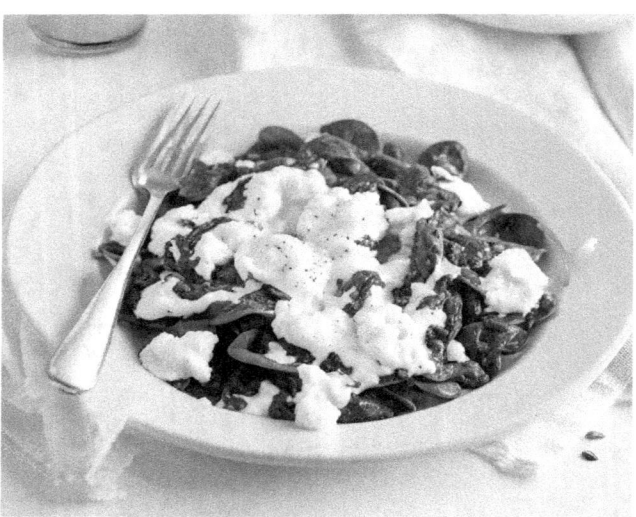

5. Zucchini and Bell Pepper Frittata

Ingredients:
- 1 small zucchini, thinly sliced
- 1 red bell pepper, chopped
- 1/2 cup chopped onions
- 6 large egg whites
- 1/4 cup low-fat milk
- 1 tablespoon olive oil
- 1/4 teaspoon garlic powder
- 1/4 teaspoon dried basil

Instructions:
1. Preheat the oven to 375°F (190°C).
2. In a non-stick, oven-safe skillet, heat olive oil over medium heat.
3. Add the chopped onions, zucchini, and red bell pepper. Sauté until vegetables are tender, about 5-7 minutes.
4. In a bowl, whisk together the egg whites, low-fat milk, garlic powder, and dried basil.
5. Pour the egg mixture over the sautéed vegetables in the skillet.
6. Cook on the stovetop for 2-3 minutes until the edges start to set.
7. Transfer the skillet to the preheated oven and bake for 10-12 minutes, or until the frittata is set.
8. Let cool for a few minutes before slicing and serving.

Nutrition Info (per serving):
- Calories: 130
- Protein: 14g
- Carbohydrates: 8g
- Fat: 5g
- Fiber: 2g
- Sugar: 5g

Serves: 2
Cooking Time: 20 minutes

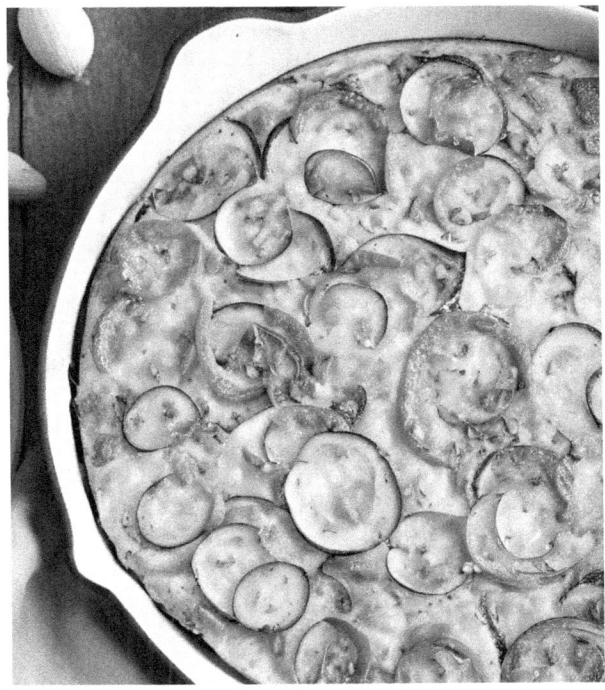

6. Apple Sauce Pancakes

Ingredients:
- 1 cup whole wheat flour
- 1 teaspoon baking powder
- 1/2 teaspoon baking soda
- 1/2 teaspoon ground cinnamon
- 1 cup unsweetened applesauce
- 1/2 cup low-fat milk
- 1 large egg
- 1 tablespoon honey (optional)
- 1 teaspoon vanilla extract
- 1 tablespoon olive oil (for cooking)

Instructions:
1. In a large bowl, combine the whole wheat flour, baking powder, baking soda, and ground cinnamon.
2. In another bowl, whisk together the applesauce, low-fat milk, egg, honey (if using), and vanilla extract.
3. Pour the wet ingredients into the dry ingredients and stir until just combined.
4. Heat a non-stick skillet or griddle over medium heat and lightly grease with olive oil.
5. Pour 1/4 cup of batter onto the skillet for each pancake.
6. Cook until bubbles form on the surface and the edges look set, about 2-3 minutes. Flip and cook for another 2-3 minutes until golden brown.
7. Serve warm.

Nutrition Info (per serving, 2 pancakes):
- Calories: 180
- Protein: 6g
- Carbohydrates: 34g
- Fat: 4g
- Fiber: 4g
- Sugar: 10g

Serves: 4 (makes 8 pancakes)
Cooking Time: 15 minutes

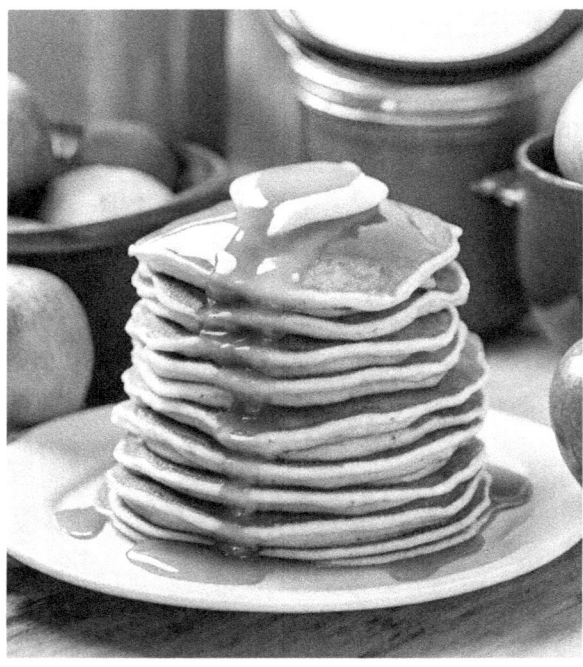

7. Baked Sweet Potato Hash

Ingredients:
- 2 medium sweet potatoes, peeled and diced
- 1 red bell pepper, chopped
- 1 green bell pepper, chopped
- 1/2 cup chopped onions
- 2 tablespoons olive oil
- 1/2 teaspoon paprika
- 1/2 teaspoon garlic powder
- 1/2 teaspoon dried thyme

Instructions:
1. Preheat the oven to 400°F (200°C).
2. In a large bowl, toss the diced sweet potatoes, bell peppers, and onions with olive oil, paprika, garlic powder, and dried thyme.
3. Spread the mixture evenly on a baking sheet.
4. Bake in the preheated oven for 25-30 minutes, stirring halfway through, until the sweet potatoes are tender and lightly browned.
5. Serve warm.

Nutrition Info (per serving):
- Calories: 180
- Protein: 3g
- Carbohydrates: 30g
- Fat: 7g
- Fiber: 5g
- Sugar: 8g

Serves: 4
Cooking Time: 30 minutes

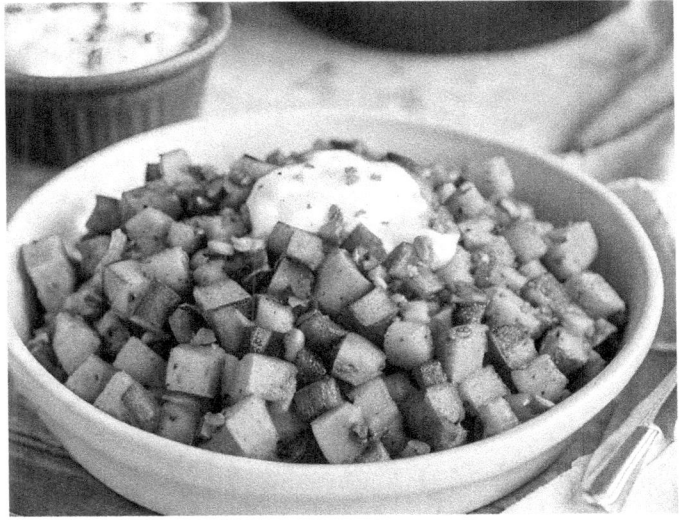

8. Peach Rice Pudding

Ingredients:
- 1 cup cooked brown rice
- 1 1/2 cups low-fat milk
- 1 cup diced peaches (fresh or canned in juice)
- 1/4 cup honey
- 1 teaspoon vanilla extract
- 1/2 teaspoon ground cinnamon
- 1/4 teaspoon ground nutmeg

Instructions:
1. In a medium saucepan, combine the cooked brown rice, low-fat milk, diced peaches, honey, vanilla extract, ground cinnamon, and ground nutmeg.
2. Bring to a simmer over medium heat, stirring occasionally.
3. Reduce heat to low and cook, stirring frequently, until the mixture thickens and becomes creamy, about 20-25 minutes.
4. Remove from heat and let cool slightly before serving. Can be served warm or chilled.

Nutrition Info (per serving):
- Calories: 220
- Protein: 6g
- Carbohydrates: 45g
- Fat: 2g
- Fiber: 3g
- Sugar: 23g

Serves: 4
Cooking Time: 30 minutes

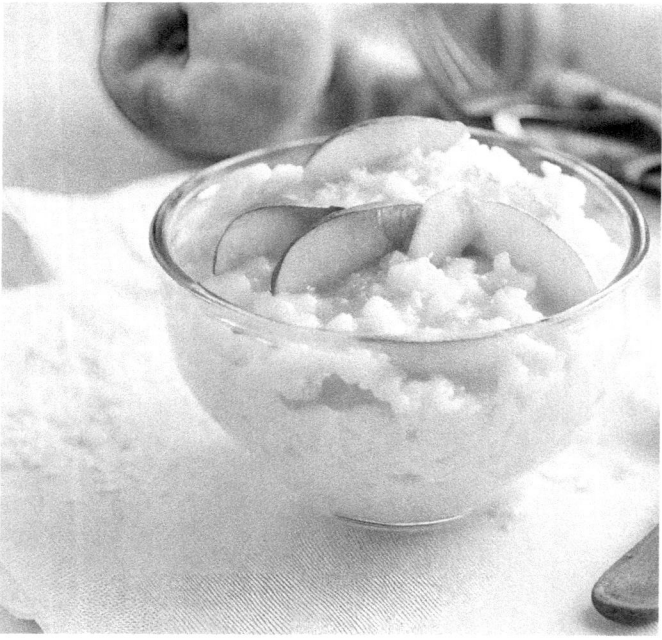

9. Savory Oatmeal with Poached Egg

Ingredients:
- 1/2 cup rolled oats
- 1 cup low-sodium vegetable broth
- 1/2 cup chopped spinach
- 1 tablespoon grated Parmesan cheese
- 1 large egg
- 1 tablespoon white vinegar
- 1/4 teaspoon garlic powder
- 1/4 teaspoon dried thyme

Instructions:
1. In a medium saucepan, bring the vegetable broth to a boil.
2. Stir in the rolled oats, garlic powder, and dried thyme. Reduce heat and simmer for 5-7 minutes, stirring occasionally.
3. Add the chopped spinach and cook for another 2 minutes until the oats are tender and the spinach is wilted.
4. Stir in the grated Parmesan cheese and remove from heat.
5. In a small saucepan, bring water to a gentle simmer and add the white vinegar.
6. Crack the egg into a small bowl and gently slide it into the simmering water.
7. Poach the egg for about 3-4 minutes until the white is set but the yolk is still runny.
8. Remove the egg with a slotted spoon and place it on top of the savory oatmeal.
9. Serve immediately.

Nutrition Info (per serving):
- Calories: 250
- Protein: 14g
- Carbohydrates: 31g
- Fat: 8g
- Fiber: 4g
- Sugar: 2g

Serves: 1
Cooking Time: 15 minutes

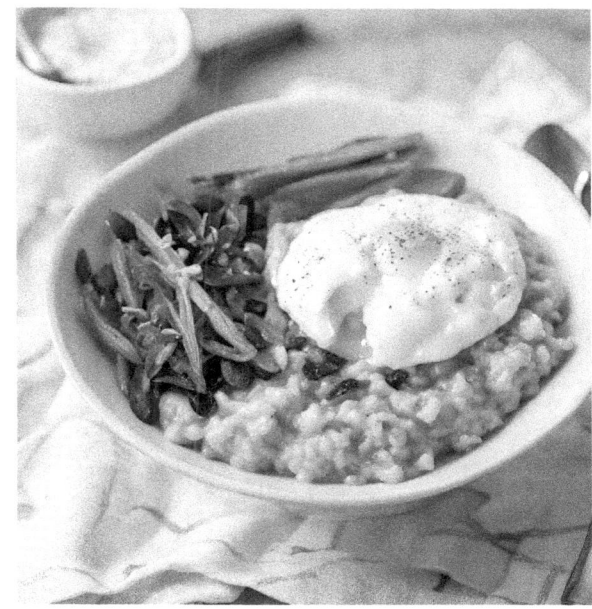

10. Pumpkin Spice Oatmeal

Ingredients:
- 1/2 cup rolled oats
- 1 cup low-fat milk or unsweetened almond milk
- 1/4 cup pumpkin puree
- 1 tablespoon honey
- 1/2 teaspoon ground cinnamon
- 1/4 teaspoon ground nutmeg
- 1/4 teaspoon ground ginger
- 1/4 teaspoon ground cloves
- 1/4 teaspoon vanilla extract

Instructions:
1. In a medium saucepan, combine the rolled oats and milk. Bring to a boil over medium heat.
2. Reduce heat and stir in the pumpkin puree, honey, ground cinnamon, nutmeg, ginger, cloves, and vanilla extract.
3. Simmer for 5-7 minutes, stirring occasionally, until the oats are tender and the mixture is creamy.
4. Remove from heat and let sit for a minute before serving.

Nutrition Info (per serving):
- Calories: 220
- Protein: 6g
- Carbohydrates: 40g
- Fat: 4g
- Fiber: 5g
- Sugar: 15g

Serves: 1
Cooking Time: 10 minutes

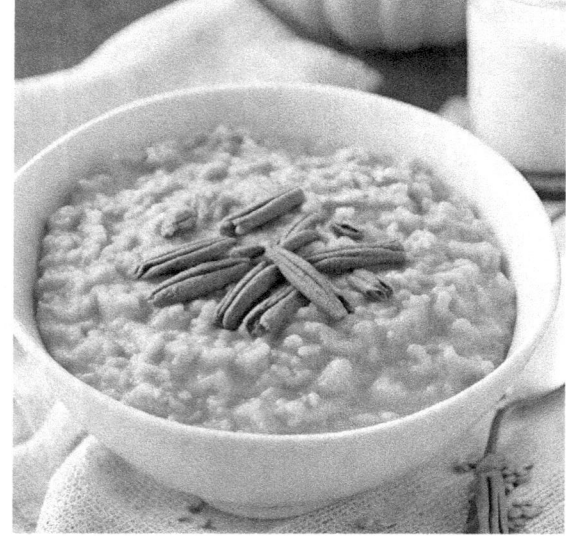

11. Herbal Tea with Rice Cakes

Ingredients:
- 1 herbal tea bag (e.g., chamomile, peppermint)
- 1 cup hot water
- 2 plain rice cakes
- 1 tablespoon almond butter
- 1/2 apple, thinly sliced

Instructions:
1. Brew the herbal tea by steeping the tea bag in hot water for 3-5 minutes.
2. Spread the almond butter evenly over the rice cakes.
3. Top each rice cake with thinly sliced apple.
4. Serve the rice cakes with the brewed herbal tea.

Nutrition Info (per serving):
- Calories: 180
- Protein: 4g
- Carbohydrates: 30g
- Fat: 6g
- Fiber: 4g
- Sugar: 10g

Serves: 1
Cooking Time: 5 minutes

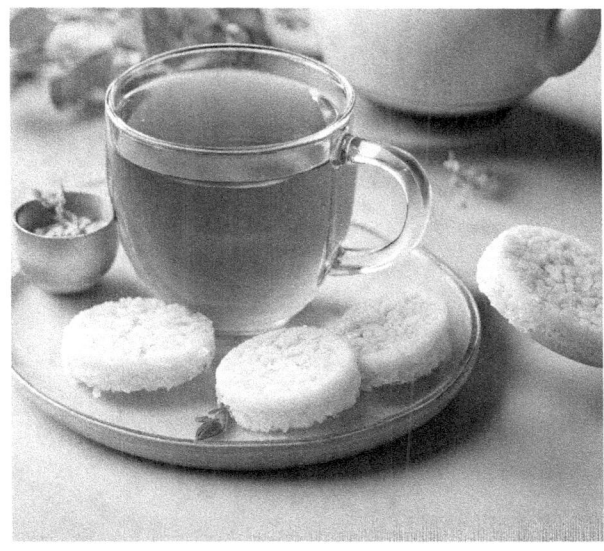

12. Almond Milk Porridge

Ingredients:
- 1/2 cup rolled oats
- 1 cup unsweetened almond milk
- 1 tablespoon chia seeds
- 1 tablespoon honey
- 1/2 teaspoon ground cinnamon
- 1/4 teaspoon vanilla extract
- 1/4 cup fresh berries (blueberries, strawberries)

Instructions:
1. In a medium saucepan, combine the rolled oats, almond milk, chia seeds, honey, ground cinnamon, and vanilla extract.
2. Bring to a boil over medium heat, then reduce heat and simmer for 5-7 minutes, stirring occasionally, until the oats are tender and the mixture is creamy.
3. Remove from heat and let sit for a minute.
4. Top with fresh berries and serve immediately.

Nutrition Info (per serving):
- Calories: 250
- Protein: 6g
- Carbohydrates: 42g
- Fat: 8g
- Fiber: 7g
- Sugar: 15g

Serves: 1
Cooking Time: 10 minutes

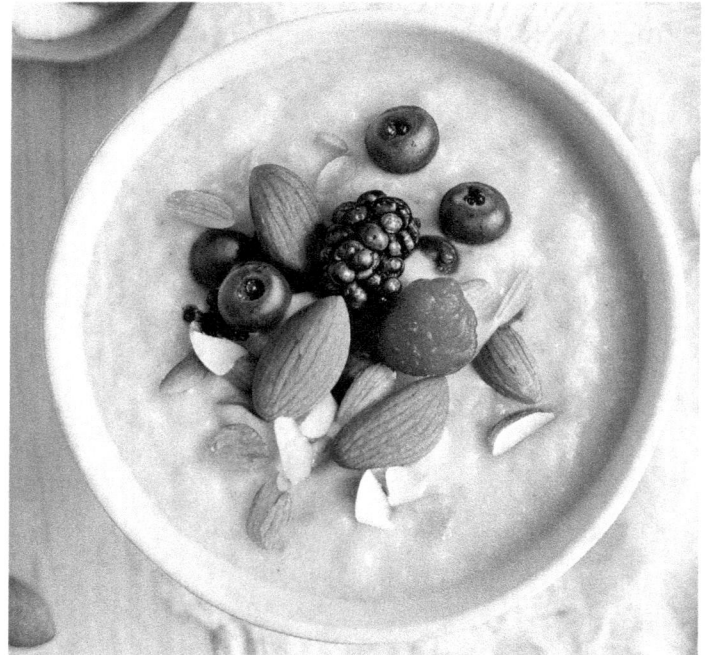

13. Buckwheat Pancakes

Ingredients:
- 1/2 cup buckwheat flour
- 1/4 cup whole wheat flour
- 1 teaspoon baking powder
- 1/2 teaspoon ground cinnamon
- 1 cup low-fat milk or unsweetened almond milk
- 1 large egg
- 1 tablespoon honey
- 1 teaspoon vanilla extract
- 1 tablespoon olive oil (for cooking)

Instructions:
1. In a large bowl, combine the buckwheat flour, whole wheat flour, baking powder, and ground cinnamon.
2. In another bowl, whisk together the milk, egg, honey, and vanilla extract.
3. Pour the wet ingredients into the dry ingredients and stir until just combined.
4. Heat a non-stick skillet or griddle over medium heat and lightly grease with olive oil.
5. Pour 1/4 cup of batter onto the skillet for each pancake.
6. Cook until bubbles form on the surface and the edges look set, about 2-3 minutes. Flip and cook for another 2-3 minutes until golden brown.
7. Serve warm.

Nutrition Info (per serving, 3 pancakes):
- Calories: 210
- Protein: 8g
- Carbohydrates: 35g
- Fat: 6g
- Fiber: 4g
- Sugar: 9g

Serves: 2 (makes 6 pancakes)
Cooking Time: 15 minutes

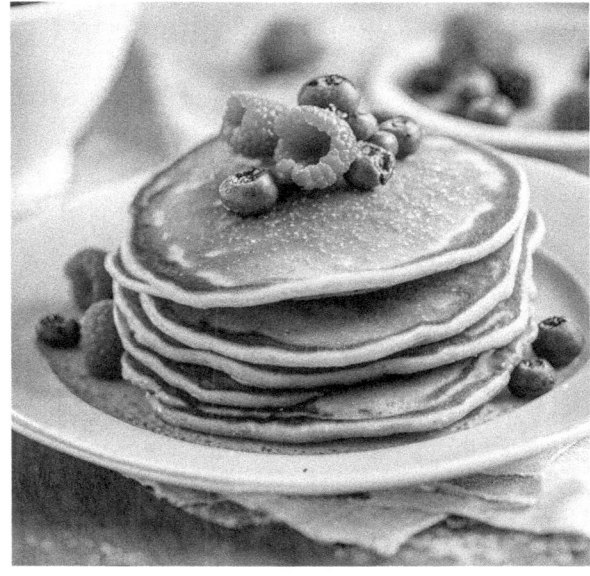

14. Steamed Vegetable Medley

Ingredients:
- 1 cup broccoli florets
- 1 cup cauliflower florets
- 1 cup baby carrots
- 1 tablespoon olive oil
- 1/4 teaspoon garlic powder
- 1/4 teaspoon dried oregano
- 1/4 teaspoon dried basil

Instructions:
1. In a large pot, bring water to a boil and place a steamer basket over the pot.
2. Add the broccoli, cauliflower, and baby carrots to the steamer basket.
3. Cover and steam the vegetables for 5-7 minutes, or until tender.
4. In a small bowl, mix the olive oil, garlic powder, dried oregano, and dried basil.
5. Drizzle the steamed vegetables with the seasoned olive oil and toss to coat evenly.
6. Serve immediately.

Nutrition Info (per serving):
- Calories: 120
- Protein: 3g
- Carbohydrates: 14g
- Fat: 7g
- Fiber: 5g
- Sugar: 6g

Serves: 2
Cooking Time: 10 minutes

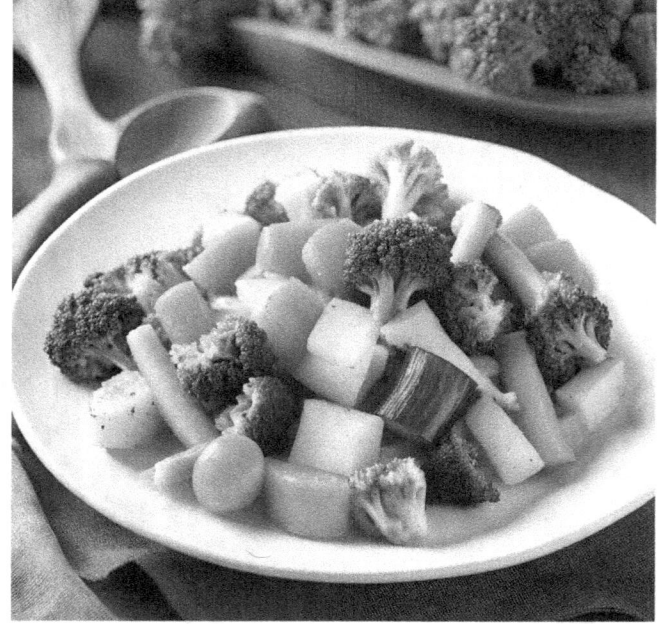

15. Pearled Barley Porridge

Ingredients:
- 1 cup pearled barley
- 4 cups water
- 1/2 cup low-fat milk or unsweetened almond milk
- 1 tablespoon honey
- 1 teaspoon vanilla extract
- 1/2 teaspoon ground cinnamon
- 1/4 cup chopped nuts (optional)

Instructions:
1. Rinse the pearled barley under cold water.
2. In a large saucepan, combine the barley and water. Bring to a boil over high heat.
3. Reduce heat to low, cover, and simmer for about 40-45 minutes, or until the barley is tender and most of the water is absorbed.
4. Stir in the milk, honey, vanilla extract, and ground cinnamon. Cook for an additional 5 minutes, stirring occasionally.
5. Remove from heat and let sit for a few minutes before serving.
6. Top with chopped nuts if desired.

Nutrition Info (per serving):
- Calories: 220
- Protein: 6g
- Carbohydrates: 44g
- Fat: 3g
- Fiber: 8g
- Sugar: 10g

Serves: 4
Cooking Time: 50 minutes

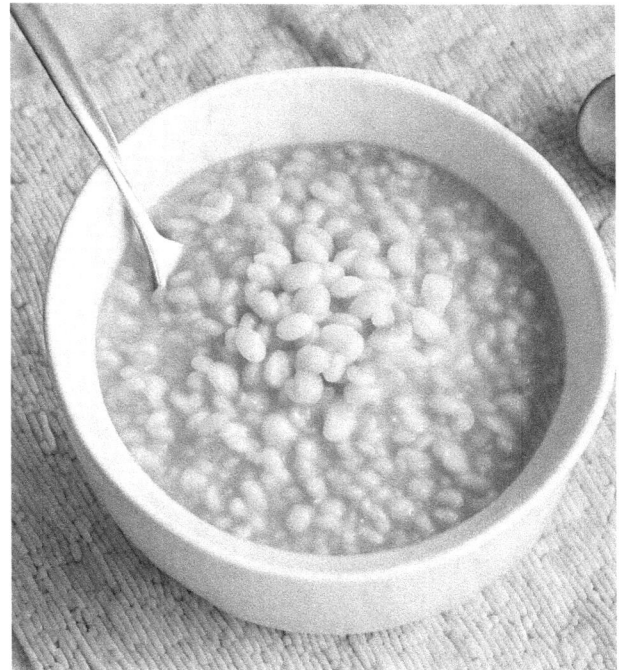

16. Banana Rice Porridge

Ingredients:
- 1 cup cooked brown rice
- 1 cup low-fat milk or unsweetened almond milk
- 1 ripe banana, mashed
- 1 tablespoon honey
- 1/2 teaspoon ground cinnamon
- 1/4 teaspoon vanilla extract
- 1 tablespoon chopped walnuts (optional)

Instructions:
1. In a medium saucepan, combine the cooked brown rice, milk, mashed banana, honey, ground cinnamon, and vanilla extract.
2. Cook over medium heat, stirring occasionally, until the mixture thickens and becomes creamy, about 10 minutes.
3. Remove from heat and let cool slightly before serving.
4. Top with chopped walnuts if desired.

Nutrition Info (per serving):
- Calories: 220
- Protein: 5g
- Carbohydrates: 42g
- Fat: 4g
- Fiber: 3g
- Sugar: 18g

Serves: 2
Cooking Time: 15 minutes

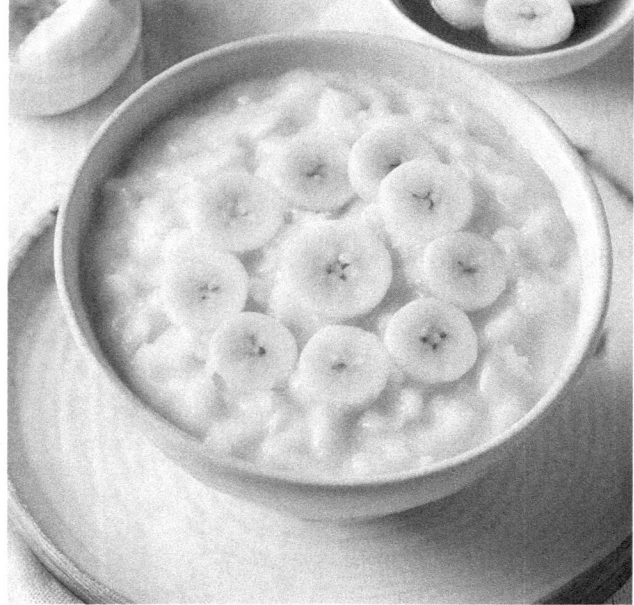

17. Egg White Omelet with Mushrooms

Ingredients:
- 4 large egg whites
- 1/2 cup chopped mushrooms
- 1/4 cup chopped onions
- 1/2 cup fresh spinach, chopped
- 1 tablespoon olive oil
- 1/4 teaspoon garlic powder
- 1/4 teaspoon dried thyme

Instructions:
1. In a bowl, whisk together the egg whites, garlic powder, and dried thyme.
2. Heat olive oil in a non-stick skillet over medium heat.
3. Add the chopped onions and mushrooms to the skillet. Sauté until tender, about 3-4 minutes.
4. Add the chopped spinach and cook until wilted, about 1-2 minutes.
5. Pour the egg white mixture over the vegetables in the skillet.
6. Cook until the eggs are set, gently folding the omelet in half, about 3-4 minutes.
7. Serve immediately.

Nutrition Info (per serving):
- Calories: 150
- Protein: 13g
- Carbohydrates: 5g
- Fat: 9g
- Fiber: 2g
- Sugar: 3g

Serves: 1
Cooking Time: 10 minutes

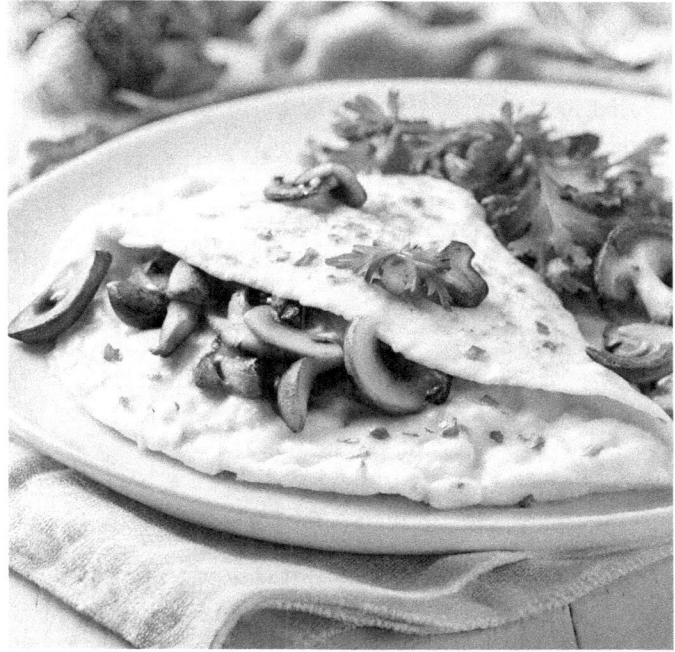

18. Quinoa and Berry Salad

Ingredients:
- 1 cup cooked quinoa
- 1/2 cup fresh strawberries, sliced
- 1/2 cup fresh blueberries
- 1/2 cup fresh raspberries
- 1 tablespoon honey
- 1 tablespoon fresh lemon juice
- 1 teaspoon lemon zest
- 1/4 cup chopped mint leaves

Instructions:
1. In a large bowl, combine the cooked quinoa, strawberries, blueberries, and raspberries.
2. In a small bowl, whisk together the honey, lemon juice, and lemon zest.
3. Pour the honey-lemon dressing over the quinoa and berries. Toss gently to combine.
4. Sprinkle with chopped mint leaves and toss again.
5. Serve immediately or refrigerate until ready to eat.

Nutrition Info (per serving):
- Calories: 200
- Protein: 5g
- Carbohydrates: 40g
- Fat: 3g
- Fiber: 6g
- Sugar: 15g

Serves: 2
Cooking Time: 15 minutes

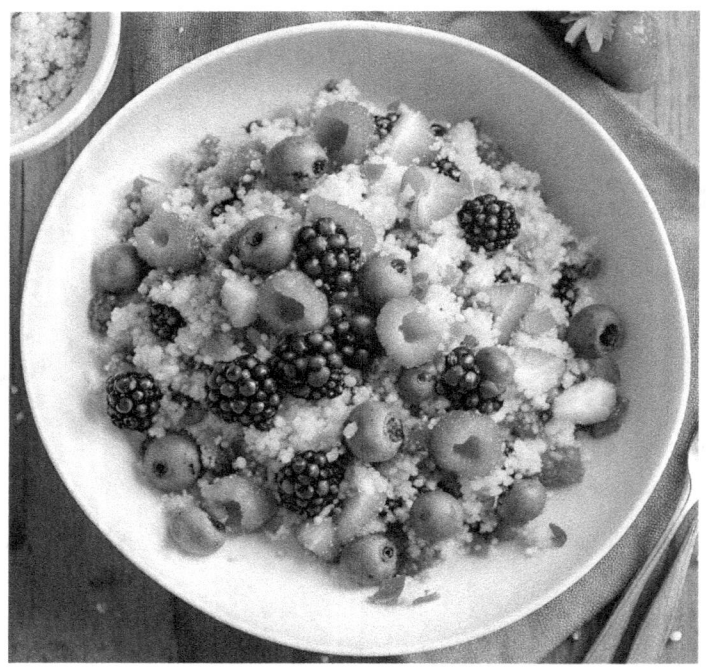

19. Sweet Potato and Kale Smoothie

Ingredients:
- 1/2 cup cooked and mashed sweet potato
- 1 cup fresh kale leaves, chopped
- 1 banana
- 1 cup unsweetened almond milk
- 1 tablespoon chia seeds
- 1 tablespoon honey
- 1/2 teaspoon ground cinnamon
- 1/2 cup ice cubes

Instructions:
1. Place the cooked sweet potato, kale, banana, almond milk, chia seeds, honey, ground cinnamon, and ice cubes in a blender.
2. Blend until smooth and creamy.
3. Pour into a glass and serve immediately.

Nutrition Info (per serving):
- Calories: 220
- Protein: 4g
- Carbohydrates: 45g
- Fat: 4g
- Fiber: 7g
- Sugar: 20g

Serves: 1
Cooking Time: 10 minutes

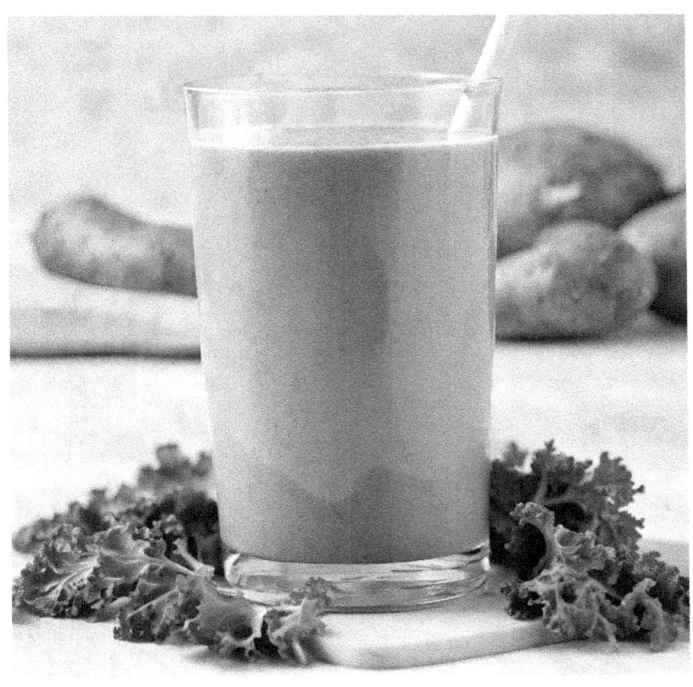

20. Carrot and Zucchini Muffins

Ingredients:
- 1 cup whole wheat flour
- 1/2 cup rolled oats
- 1 teaspoon baking powder
- 1/2 teaspoon baking soda
- 1 teaspoon ground cinnamon
- 1/2 teaspoon ground nutmeg
- 1/2 cup grated carrot
- 1/2 cup grated zucchini
- 1/2 cup unsweetened applesauce
- 1/4 cup honey
- 1/4 cup low-fat milk or unsweetened almond milk
- 1 large egg
- 1 teaspoon vanilla extract

Instructions:
1. Preheat the oven to 350°F (175°C). Line a muffin tin with paper liners or lightly grease with olive oil.
2. In a large bowl, whisk together the whole wheat flour, rolled oats, baking powder, baking soda, ground cinnamon, and ground nutmeg.
3. In another bowl, mix the grated carrot, grated zucchini, applesauce, honey, milk, egg, and vanilla extract.
4. Pour the wet ingredients into the dry ingredients and stir until just combined.
5. Divide the batter evenly among the muffin cups.
6. Bake for 18-20 minutes, or until a toothpick inserted into the center of a muffin comes out clean.
7. Let cool in the tin for a few minutes before transferring to a wire rack to cool completely.

Nutrition Info (per serving, 1 muffin):
- Calories: 130
- Protein: 3g
- Carbohydrates: 26g
- Fat: 2g
- Fiber: 3g
- Sugar: 12g

Serves: 12 muffins
Cooking Time: 25 minutes

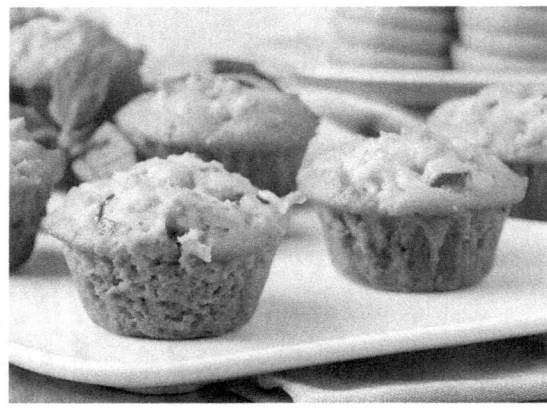

21. Squash and Apple Bake

Ingredients:
- 2 cups butternut squash, peeled and cubed
- 2 apples, peeled, cored, and sliced
- 1/4 cup raisins
- 1/4 cup honey
- 1 teaspoon ground cinnamon
- 1/2 teaspoon ground nutmeg
- 1 tablespoon olive oil

Instructions:
1. Preheat the oven to 375°F (190°C).
2. In a large mixing bowl, combine the butternut squash, apples, raisins, honey, ground cinnamon, and ground nutmeg. Toss to coat evenly.
3. Transfer the mixture to a baking dish and drizzle with olive oil.
4. Cover the dish with aluminum foil and bake for 25-30 minutes, or until the squash and apples are tender.
5. Remove the foil and bake for an additional 5 minutes to lightly brown the top.
6. Serve warm.

Nutrition Info (per serving):
- Calories: 180
- Protein: 1g
- Carbohydrates: 42g
- Fat: 3g
- Fiber: 4g
- Sugar: 30g

Serves: 4
Cooking Time: 35 minutes

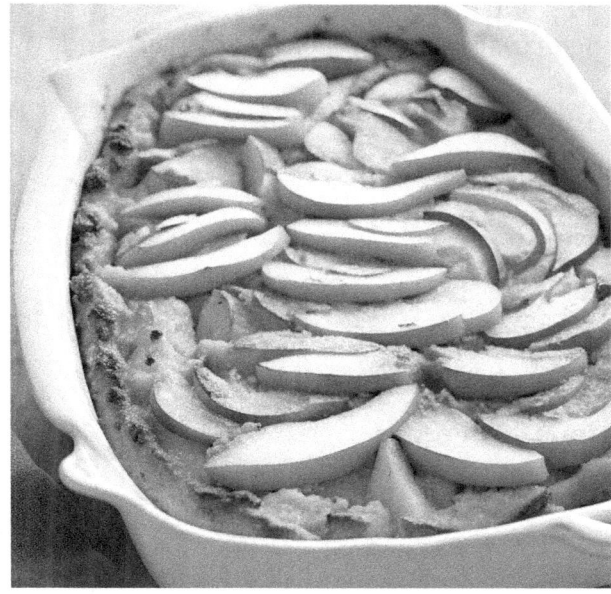

22. Warm Barley and Pumpkin Salad

Ingredients:
- 1 cup pearled barley
- 2 cups water
- 1 cup pumpkin puree
- 1/4 cup chopped walnuts
- 1/4 cup dried cranberries
- 2 tablespoons olive oil
- 1 tablespoon honey
- 1 tablespoon balsamic vinegar
- 1/2 teaspoon ground cinnamon
- 1/4 teaspoon ground ginger

Instructions:
1. Rinse the pearled barley under cold water.
2. In a medium saucepan, bring the barley and water to a boil.
3. Reduce heat to low, cover, and simmer for 25-30 minutes, or until the barley is tender and the water is absorbed.
4. In a large mixing bowl, combine the cooked barley, pumpkin puree, chopped walnuts, and dried cranberries.
5. In a small bowl, whisk together the olive oil, honey, balsamic vinegar, ground cinnamon, and ground ginger.
6. Pour the dressing over the barley mixture and toss to coat evenly.
7. Serve warm.

Nutrition Info (per serving):
- Calories: 250
- Protein: 5g
- Carbohydrates: 42g
- Fat: 9g
- Fiber: 7g
- Sugar: 15g

Serves: 4
Cooking Time: 35 minutes

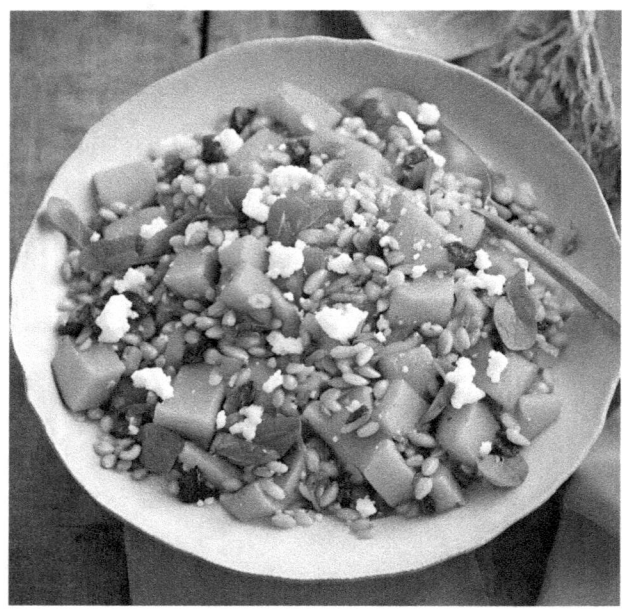

23. Tapioca Pudding

Ingredients:
- 1/2 cup small pearl tapioca
- 2 1/2 cups low-fat milk or unsweetened almond milk
- 1/4 cup honey
- 1 teaspoon vanilla extract
- 1/2 teaspoon ground cinnamon
- 1/4 teaspoon ground nutmeg

Instructions:
1. In a medium saucepan, combine the tapioca and milk. Let it sit for 30 minutes to soak.
2. Place the saucepan over medium heat and bring to a gentle boil, stirring frequently.
3. Reduce heat to low and simmer, stirring often, until the tapioca pearls are transparent and the mixture thickens, about 20-25 minutes.
4. Remove from heat and stir in the honey, vanilla extract, ground cinnamon, and ground nutmeg.
5. Let cool slightly before serving. Can be served warm or chilled.

Nutrition Info (per serving):
- Calories: 180
- Protein: 4g
- Carbohydrates: 35g
- Fat: 3g
- Fiber: 1g
- Sugar: 20g

Serves: 4
Cooking Time: 60 minutes (including soaking time)

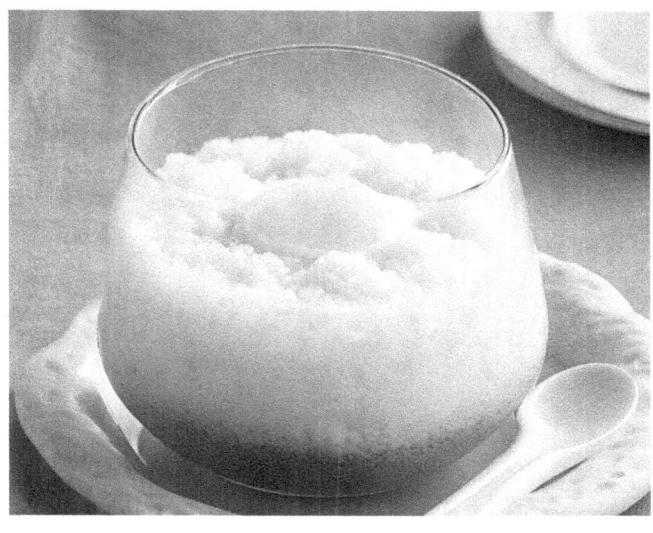

Fish & Seafood Recipes

1. Poached Cod with Parsley and Lemon

Ingredients:
- 4 cod fillets (about 6 ounces each)
- 4 cups low-sodium vegetable broth
- 1 lemon, thinly sliced
- 1/4 cup fresh parsley, chopped
- 2 cloves garlic, minced
- 1 tablespoon olive oil
- 1/2 teaspoon dried thyme

Instructions:
1. In a large skillet, bring the vegetable broth to a simmer over medium heat.
2. Add the lemon slices, garlic, and dried thyme to the skillet.
3. Carefully place the cod fillets into the simmering broth.
4. Cover and poach the fish for 8-10 minutes, or until the cod is opaque and flakes easily with a fork.
5. Remove the cod from the skillet and place on serving plates.
6. Drizzle with olive oil and sprinkle with fresh parsley.
7. Serve immediately with lemon slices.

Nutrition Info (per serving):
- Calories: 220
- Protein: 34g
- Carbohydrates: 4g
- Fat: 8g
- Fiber: 1g
- Sugar: 1g

Serves: 4
Cooking Time: 15 minutes

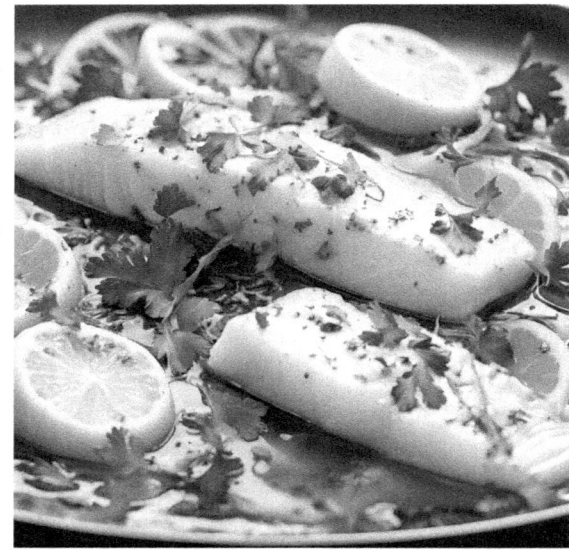

2. Steamed Clams in White Wine

Ingredients:
- 2 pounds fresh clams, scrubbed
- 1 cup low-sodium vegetable broth
- 1 cup dry white wine
- 2 cloves garlic, minced
- 1 shallot, finely chopped
- 1 tablespoon olive oil
- 1/4 cup fresh parsley, chopped
- 1/2 teaspoon dried oregano
- 1/2 teaspoon ground black pepper

Instructions:
1. In a large pot, heat the olive oil over medium heat.
2. Add the garlic and shallot, and sauté for 2-3 minutes until fragrant and translucent.
3. Pour in the vegetable broth and white wine, and bring to a simmer.
4. Add the clams, cover the pot, and steam for 5-7 minutes, or until the clams open. Discard any clams that do not open.
5. Remove the clams from the pot and place in a large serving bowl.
6. Stir in the dried oregano and ground black pepper into the broth.
7. Pour the broth over the clams and sprinkle with fresh parsley.
8. Serve immediately.

Nutrition Info (per serving):
- Calories: 200
- Protein: 25g
- Carbohydrates: 7g
- Fat: 4g
- Fiber: 1g
- Sugar: 2g

Serves: 4
Cooking Time: 15 minutes

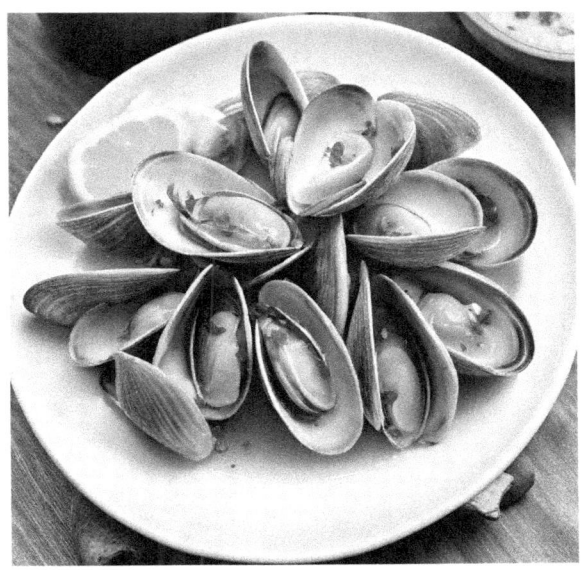

3. Grilled Tilapia with Herbs

Ingredients:
- 4 tilapia fillets (about 6 ounces each)
- 2 tablespoons olive oil
- 2 cloves garlic, minced
- 1 tablespoon fresh lemon juice
- 1 teaspoon dried basil
- 1 teaspoon dried oregano
- 1/2 teaspoon ground black pepper
- 1/4 cup fresh parsley, chopped

Instructions:
1. Preheat the grill to medium-high heat.
2. In a small bowl, combine the olive oil, garlic, lemon juice, dried basil, dried oregano, and ground black pepper.
3. Brush both sides of the tilapia fillets with the olive oil mixture.
4. Place the tilapia on the preheated grill and cook for 3-4 minutes per side, or until the fish is opaque and flakes easily with a fork.
5. Remove from the grill and sprinkle with fresh parsley.
6. Serve immediately.

Nutrition Info (per serving):
- Calories: 210
- Protein: 35g
- Carbohydrates: 2g
- Fat: 7g
- Fiber: 1g
- Sugar: 1g

Serves: 4
Cooking Time: 10 minutes

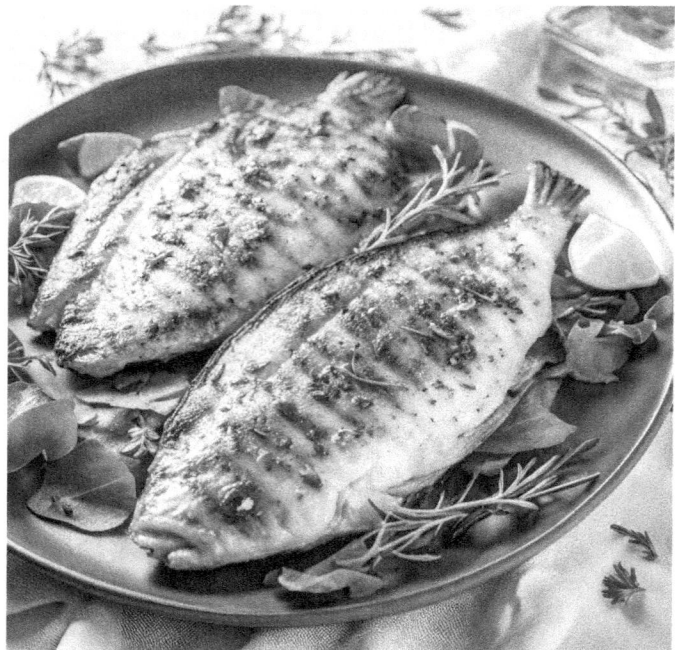

4. Baked Sole with Dill

Ingredients:
- 4 sole fillets (about 6 ounces each)
- 1 lemon, thinly sliced
- 1/4 cup fresh dill, chopped
- 2 cloves garlic, minced
- 1 tablespoon olive oil
- 1/4 teaspoon ground black pepper

Instructions:
1. Preheat the oven to 375°F (190°C).
2. In a small bowl, combine the olive oil, garlic, and ground black pepper.
3. Arrange the sole fillets in a baking dish.
4. Brush the fillets with the olive oil mixture.
5. Top each fillet with lemon slices and sprinkle with fresh dill.
6. Cover the baking dish with aluminum foil and bake for 15-20 minutes, or until the fish is opaque and flakes easily with a fork.
7. Remove from the oven and serve immediately.

Nutrition Info (per serving):
- Calories: 190
- Protein: 33g
- Carbohydrates: 2g
- Fat: 5g
- Fiber: 1g
- Sugar: 1g

Serves: 4
Cooking Time: 20 minutes

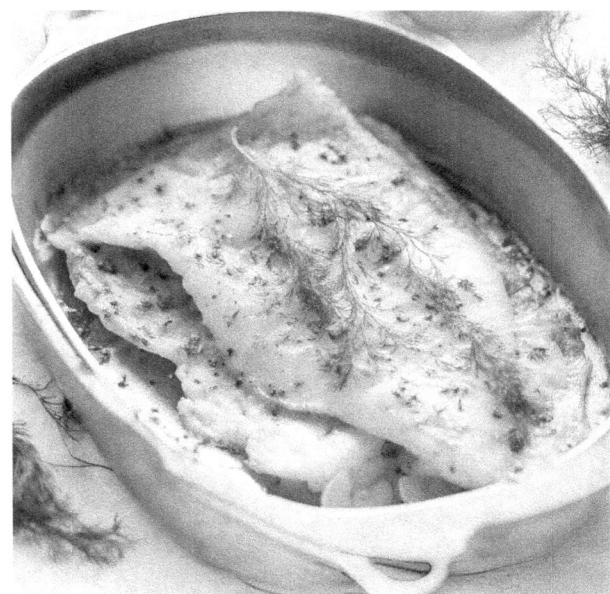

5. Shrimp and Cucumber Salad

Ingredients:
- 1 pound cooked shrimp, peeled and deveined
- 2 cucumbers, thinly sliced
- 1/4 cup red onion, thinly sliced
- 1/4 cup fresh dill, chopped
- 1/4 cup olive oil
- 2 tablespoons fresh lemon juice
- 1 teaspoon Dijon mustard
- 1/2 teaspoon ground black pepper

Instructions:
1. In a large bowl, combine the cooked shrimp, sliced cucumbers, red onion, and fresh dill.
2. In a small bowl, whisk together the olive oil, lemon juice, Dijon mustard, and ground black pepper.
3. Pour the dressing over the shrimp and cucumber mixture and toss to coat evenly.
4. Serve immediately or refrigerate until ready to serve.

Nutrition Info (per serving):
- Calories: 220
- Protein: 23g
- Carbohydrates: 5g
- Fat: 12g
- Fiber: 1g
- Sugar: 2g

Serves: 4
Cooking Time: 10 minutes

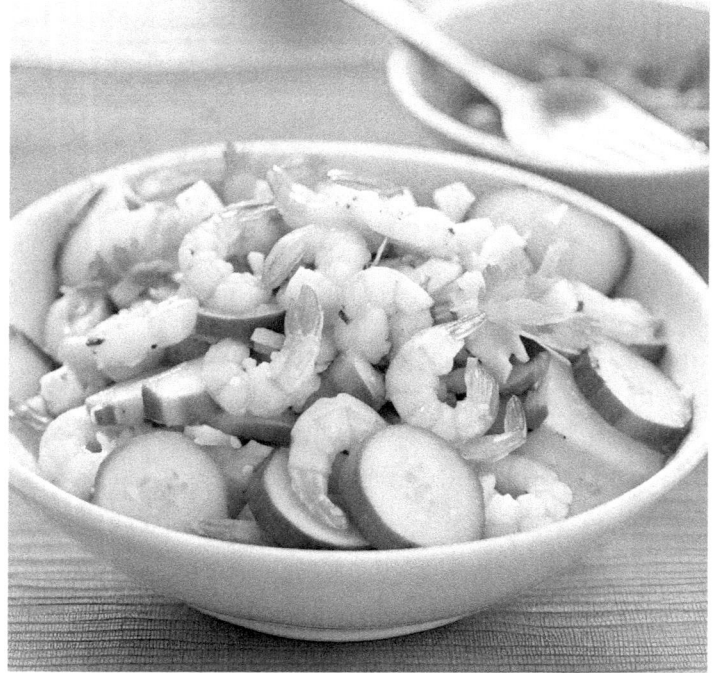

6. Seared Scallops with Lemon Zest

Ingredients:
- 1 pound sea scallops
- 2 tablespoons olive oil
- 2 cloves garlic, minced
- 1 lemon, zested and juiced
- 1/4 cup fresh parsley, chopped
- 1/2 teaspoon ground black pepper

Instructions:
1. Pat the scallops dry with a paper towel and season with ground black pepper.
2. Heat olive oil in a large skillet over medium-high heat.
3. Add the minced garlic and sauté for 1 minute until fragrant.
4. Add the scallops to the skillet and sear for 2-3 minutes on each side until golden brown and cooked through.
5. Remove the scallops from the skillet and place on a serving plate.
6. Drizzle with lemon juice and sprinkle with lemon zest and fresh parsley.
7. Serve immediately.

Nutrition Info (per serving):
- Calories: 200
- Protein: 25g
- Carbohydrates: 4g
- Fat: 10g
- Fiber: 1g
- Sugar: 1g

Serves: 4
Cooking Time: 10 minutes

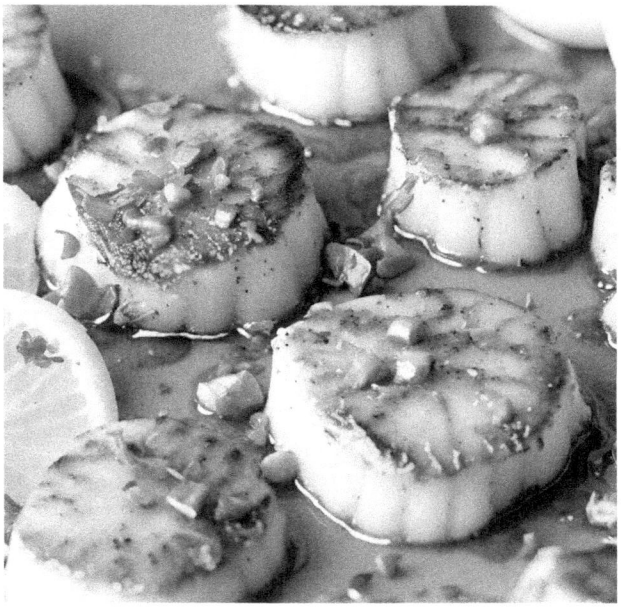

7. Broiled Haddock with Rosemary

Ingredients:
- 4 haddock fillets (about 6 ounces each)
- 2 tablespoons olive oil
- 2 cloves garlic, minced
- 1 teaspoon dried rosemary
- 1 lemon, thinly sliced
- 1/4 teaspoon ground black pepper

Instructions:
1. Preheat the broiler.
2. In a small bowl, combine the olive oil, minced garlic, dried rosemary, and ground black pepper.
3. Brush both sides of the haddock fillets with the olive oil mixture.
4. Place the haddock fillets on a broiler pan and top with lemon slices.
5. Broil for 8-10 minutes, or until the fish is opaque and flakes easily with a fork.
6. Serve immediately.

Nutrition Info (per serving):
- Calories: 210
- Protein: 35g
- Carbohydrates: 2g
- Fat: 7g
- Fiber: 1g
- Sugar: 1g

Serves: 4
Cooking Time: 10 minutes

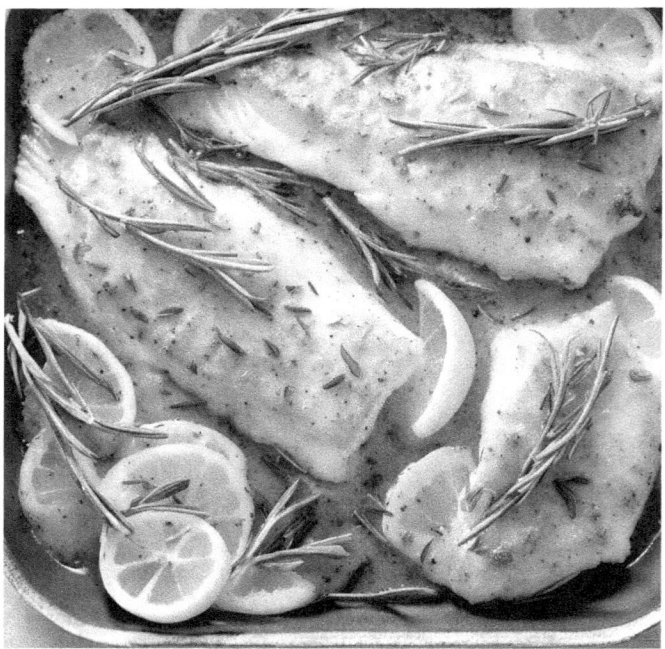

8. Herb Marinated Grilled Shrimp

Ingredients:
- 1 pound large shrimp, peeled and deveined
- 1/4 cup olive oil
- 2 tablespoons fresh lemon juice
- 2 cloves garlic, minced
- 1 tablespoon fresh thyme, chopped
- 1 tablespoon fresh rosemary, chopped
- 1/2 teaspoon ground black pepper

Instructions:
1. In a large bowl, whisk together the olive oil, lemon juice, minced garlic, fresh thyme, fresh rosemary, and ground black pepper.
2. Add the shrimp to the bowl and toss to coat evenly.
3. Cover and marinate in the refrigerator for at least 30 minutes.
4. Preheat the grill to medium-high heat.
5. Thread the shrimp onto skewers.
6. Grill the shrimp for 2-3 minutes on each side, or until pink and opaque.
7. Remove from the grill and serve immediately.

Nutrition Info (per serving):
- Calories: 220
- Protein: 24g
- Carbohydrates: 2g
- Fat: 14g
- Fiber: 1g
- Sugar: 1g

Serves: 4

Cooking Time: 10 minutes (plus marinating time)

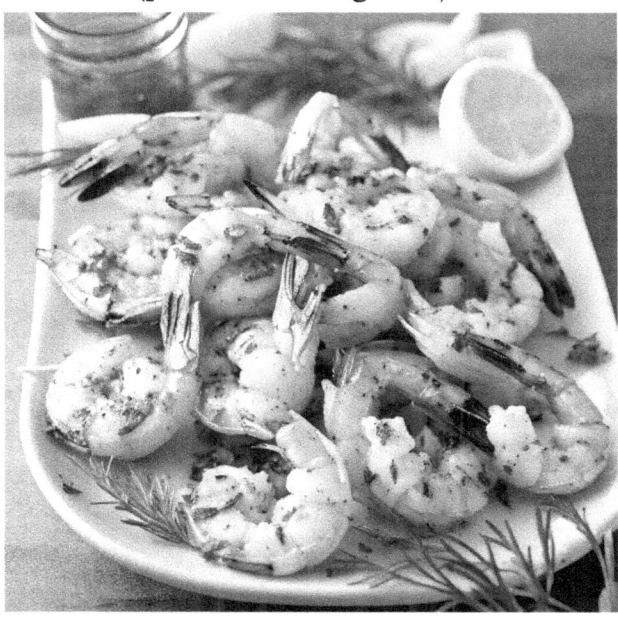

9. Ginger Soy Glazed Salmon

Ingredients:
- 4 salmon fillets (about 6 ounces each)
- 1/4 cup low-sodium soy sauce
- 2 tablespoons honey
- 1 tablespoon fresh ginger, grated
- 2 cloves garlic, minced
- 1 tablespoon olive oil
- 1/4 teaspoon ground black pepper
- 1 green onion, sliced (for garnish)

Instructions:
1. In a small bowl, whisk together the soy sauce, honey, grated ginger, minced garlic, olive oil, and ground black pepper.
2. Place the salmon fillets in a shallow dish and pour the marinade over them. Cover and marinate in the refrigerator for at least 30 minutes.
3. Preheat the oven to 375°F (190°C).
4. Line a baking sheet with parchment paper and place the salmon fillets on the sheet.
5. Bake for 15-20 minutes, or until the salmon is cooked through and flakes easily with a fork.
6. Garnish with sliced green onion and serve immediately.

Nutrition Info (per serving):
- Calories: 300
- Protein: 30g
- Carbohydrates: 10g
- Fat: 16g
- Fiber: 1g
- Sugar: 7g

Serves: 4
Cooking Time: 20 minutes (plus marinating time)

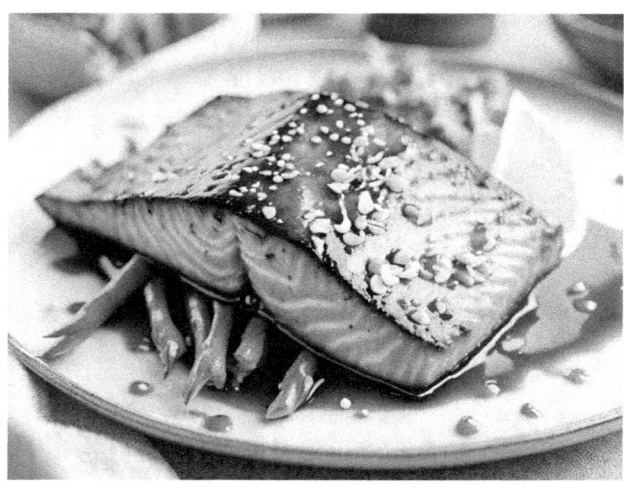

10. Poached Trout with Mint

Ingredients:
- 4 trout fillets (about 6 ounces each)
- 4 cups low-sodium vegetable broth
- 1/4 cup fresh mint leaves, chopped
- 1 lemon, thinly sliced
- 2 cloves garlic, minced
- 1 tablespoon olive oil
- 1/2 teaspoon ground black pepper

Instructions:
1. In a large skillet, bring the vegetable broth to a simmer over medium heat.
2. Add the lemon slices, garlic, and ground black pepper to the skillet.
3. Carefully place the trout fillets into the simmering broth.
4. Cover and poach the fish for 8-10 minutes, or until the trout is opaque and flakes easily with a fork.
5. Remove the trout from the skillet and place on serving plates.
6. Drizzle with olive oil and sprinkle with fresh mint.
7. Serve immediately with lemon slices.

Nutrition Info (per serving):
- Calories: 230
- Protein: 34g
- Carbohydrates: 4g
- Fat: 8g
- Fiber: 1g
- Sugar: 1g

Serves: 4
Cooking Time: 15 minutes

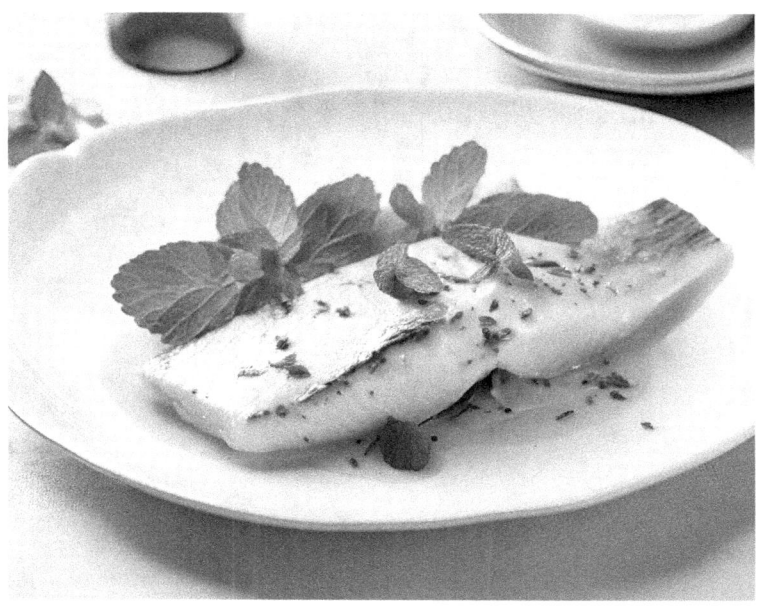

11. Mussels Steamed in Tomato Broth

Ingredients:
- 2 pounds fresh mussels, scrubbed and debearded
- 1 cup low-sodium vegetable broth
- 1 cup diced tomatoes (canned, no added salt)
- 1/2 cup dry white wine
- 2 cloves garlic, minced
- 1 shallot, finely chopped
- 1 tablespoon olive oil
- 1/4 cup fresh parsley, chopped
- 1/2 teaspoon dried oregano

Instructions:
1. In a large pot, heat the olive oil over medium heat.
2. Add the garlic and shallot, and sauté for 2-3 minutes until fragrant and translucent.
3. Add the diced tomatoes, vegetable broth, and white wine, and bring to a simmer.
4. Add the mussels, cover the pot, and steam for 5-7 minutes, or until the mussels open. Discard any mussels that do not open.
5. Remove the mussels from the pot and place in a large serving bowl.
6. Stir the dried oregano into the tomato broth.
7. Pour the broth over the mussels and sprinkle with fresh parsley.
8. Serve immediately.

Nutrition Info (per serving):
- Calories: 210
- Protein: 26g
- Carbohydrates: 8g
- Fat: 5g
- Fiber: 2g
- Sugar: 3g

Serves: 4
Cooking Time: 15 minutes

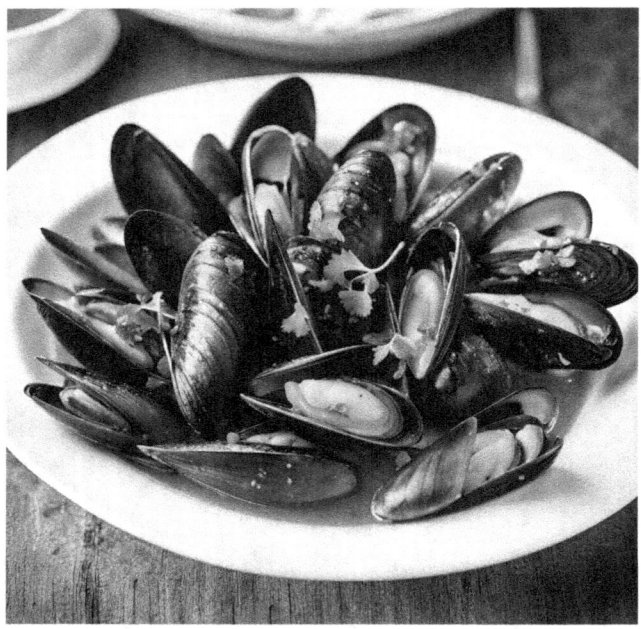

12. Lemon Garlic Tilapia

Ingredients:
- 4 tilapia fillets (about 6 ounces each)
- 2 tablespoons olive oil
- 2 cloves garlic, minced
- 1 lemon, thinly sliced
- 1 tablespoon fresh lemon juice
- 1/2 teaspoon dried basil
- 1/2 teaspoon ground black pepper

Instructions:
1. Preheat the oven to 375°F (190°C).
2. In a small bowl, combine the olive oil, minced garlic, lemon juice, dried basil, and ground black pepper.
3. Place the tilapia fillets in a baking dish.
4. Brush both sides of the tilapia fillets with the olive oil mixture.
5. Top each fillet with lemon slices.
6. Bake for 15-20 minutes, or until the fish is opaque and flakes easily with a fork.
7. Serve immediately.

Nutrition Info (per serving):
- Calories: 200
- Protein: 35g
- Carbohydrates: 2g
- Fat: 7g
- Fiber: 1g
- Sugar: 1g

Serves: 4
Cooking Time: 20 minutes

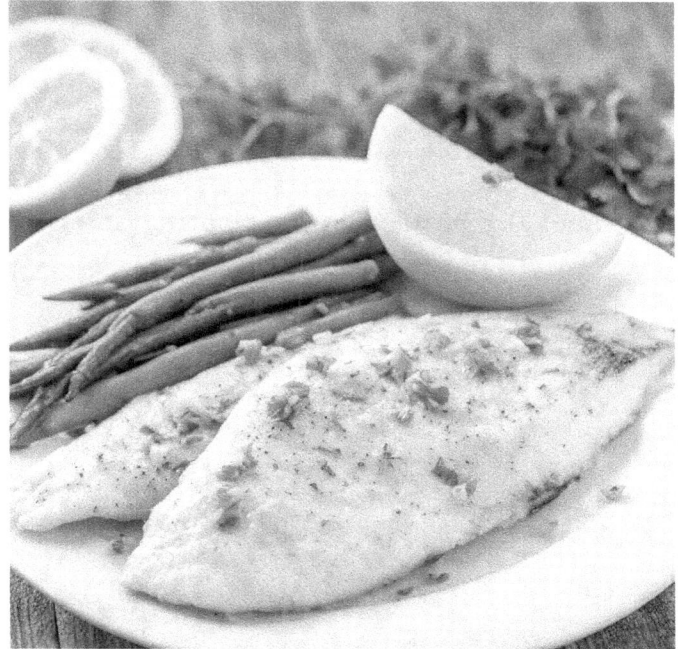

13. Orange-Rosemary Seared Salmon

Ingredients:
- 4 salmon fillets (about 6 ounces each)
- 1/4 cup fresh orange juice
- 1 tablespoon orange zest
- 2 tablespoons olive oil
- 1 tablespoon fresh rosemary, chopped
- 2 cloves garlic, minced
- 1/2 teaspoon ground black pepper

Instructions:
1. In a small bowl, whisk together the orange juice, orange zest, olive oil, fresh rosemary, minced garlic, and ground black pepper.
2. Place the salmon fillets in a shallow dish and pour the marinade over them. Cover and marinate in the refrigerator for at least 30 minutes.
3. Heat a non-stick skillet over medium-high heat.
4. Remove the salmon fillets from the marinade and place them in the skillet.
5. Sear the salmon for 4-5 minutes on each side, or until the fish is cooked through and flakes easily with a fork.
6. Serve immediately.

Nutrition Info (per serving):
- Calories: 320
- Protein: 30g
- Carbohydrates: 4g
- Fat: 20g
- Fiber: 1g
- Sugar: 2g

Serves: 4
Cooking Time: 10 minutes (plus marinating time)

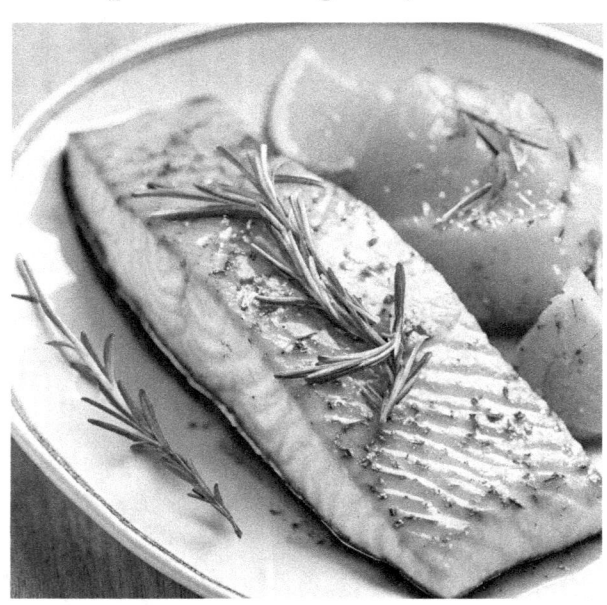

14. Prawn Stir Fry with Bell Peppers

Ingredients:
- 1 pound large prawns, peeled and deveined
- 1 red bell pepper, sliced
- 1 yellow bell pepper, sliced
- 1 green bell pepper, sliced
- 1/2 cup snow peas
- 2 tablespoons olive oil
- 2 cloves garlic, minced
- 1 tablespoon fresh ginger, grated
- 2 tablespoons low-sodium soy sauce
- 1 tablespoon fresh lime juice

Instructions:
1. Heat the olive oil in a large skillet or wok over medium-high heat.
2. Add the garlic and ginger, and sauté for 1-2 minutes until fragrant.
3. Add the sliced bell peppers and snow peas, and stir-fry for 3-4 minutes until tender-crisp.
4. Add the prawns to the skillet and cook for another 3-4 minutes until they turn pink and opaque.
5. Stir in the soy sauce and lime juice, and cook for another 1-2 minutes.
6. Serve immediately.

Nutrition Info (per serving):
- Calories: 230
- Protein: 26g
- Carbohydrates: 10g
- Fat: 10g
- Fiber: 3g
- Sugar: 4g

Serves: 4
Cooking Time: 10 minutes

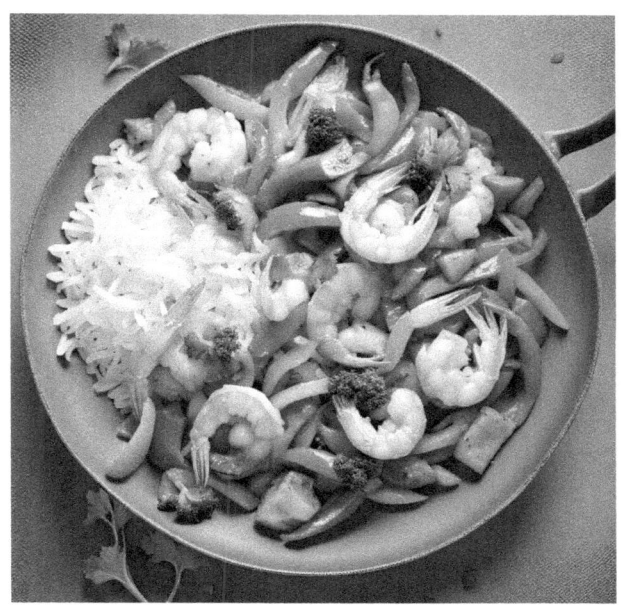

15. Flounder with Tomato Basil Sauce

Ingredients:
- 4 flounder fillets (about 6 ounces each)
- 2 tablespoons olive oil
- 2 cloves garlic, minced
- 1 cup diced tomatoes (canned, no added salt)
- 1/4 cup fresh basil, chopped
- 1 tablespoon fresh lemon juice
- 1/2 teaspoon ground black pepper

Instructions:
1. Preheat the oven to 375°F (190°C).
2. In a small skillet, heat the olive oil over medium heat.
3. Add the minced garlic and sauté for 1-2 minutes until fragrant.
4. Stir in the diced tomatoes, fresh basil, lemon juice, and ground black pepper. Simmer for 5 minutes.
5. Place the flounder fillets in a baking dish.
6. Pour the tomato basil sauce over the flounder fillets.
7. Bake for 15-20 minutes, or until the fish is opaque and flakes easily with a fork.
8. Serve immediately.

Nutrition Info (per serving):
- Calories: 210
- Protein: 34g
- Carbohydrates: 6g
- Fat: 7g
- Fiber: 2g
- Sugar: 3g

Serves: 4
Cooking Time: 20 minutes

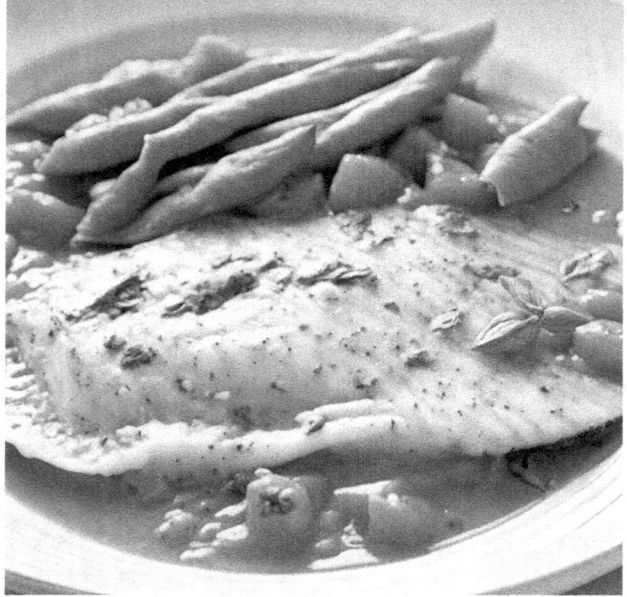

16. Seafood Paella with Brown Rice

Ingredients:
- 1 cup brown rice
- 2 cups low-sodium vegetable broth
- 1 tablespoon olive oil
- 1 onion, finely chopped
- 2 cloves garlic, minced
- 1 red bell pepper, chopped
- 1/2 teaspoon ground turmeric
- 1/2 teaspoon smoked paprika
- 1/2 pound shrimp, peeled and deveined
- 1/2 pound mussels, scrubbed and debearded
- 1/2 pound squid rings
- 1/2 cup frozen peas
- 1 lemon, cut into wedges
- 1/4 cup fresh parsley, chopped

Instructions:
1. In a large pan, heat the olive oil over medium heat. Add the onion and garlic, and sauté for 2-3 minutes until fragrant.
2. Add the red bell pepper and cook for another 2 minutes.
3. Stir in the brown rice, ground turmeric, and smoked paprika. Cook for 1 minute.
4. Pour in the vegetable broth and bring to a boil. Reduce heat to low, cover, and simmer for 40 minutes or until the rice is tender.
5. Add the shrimp, mussels, squid rings, and frozen peas. Cover and cook for another 10 minutes, or until the seafood is cooked through and the mussels have opened.
6. Remove from heat and let stand for 5 minutes.
7. Garnish with lemon wedges and fresh parsley before serving.

Nutrition Info (per serving):
- Calories: 350
- Protein: 28g
- Carbohydrates: 45g
- Fat: 9g
- Fiber: 5g
- Sugar: 4g

Serves: 4
Cooking Time: 60 minutes

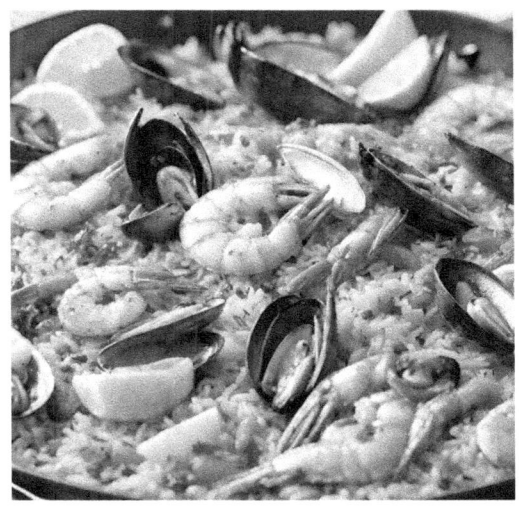

17. Asian-Style Steamed Fish

Ingredients:
- 4 white fish fillets (such as cod or snapper, about 6 ounces each)
- 2 tablespoons low-sodium soy sauce
- 1 tablespoon fresh lime juice
- 1 tablespoon fresh ginger, grated
- 2 cloves garlic, minced
- 2 green onions, sliced
- 1 tablespoon sesame oil
- 1/4 cup fresh cilantro, chopped

Instructions:
1. In a small bowl, whisk together the soy sauce, lime juice, ginger, and garlic.
2. Place the fish fillets in a shallow dish and pour the marinade over them. Let marinate for 15 minutes.
3. In a steamer, bring water to a boil. Place the fish fillets in the steamer basket and drizzle with sesame oil.
4. Cover and steam for 10-12 minutes, or until the fish is opaque and flakes easily with a fork.
5. Remove the fish from the steamer and place on serving plates.
6. Garnish with sliced green onions and fresh cilantro.
7. Serve immediately.

Nutrition Info (per serving):
- Calories: 220
- Protein: 32g
- Carbohydrates: 2g
- Fat: 9g
- Fiber: 1g
- Sugar: 1g

Serves: 4

Cooking Time: 20 minutes (plus marinating time)

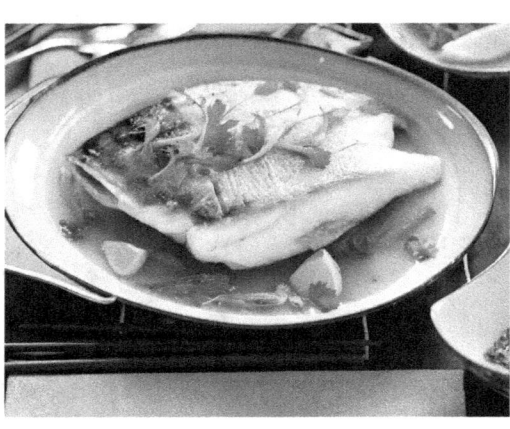

18. Cajun Seasoned Grilled Trout

Ingredients:
- 4 trout fillets (about 6 ounces each)
- 2 tablespoons olive oil
- 1 tablespoon Cajun seasoning
- 2 cloves garlic, minced
- 1 lemon, thinly sliced
- 1/4 cup fresh parsley, chopped

Instructions:
1. Preheat the grill to medium-high heat.
2. In a small bowl, combine the olive oil, Cajun seasoning, and minced garlic.
3. Brush both sides of the trout fillets with the olive oil mixture.
4. Place the trout fillets on the preheated grill and cook for 4-5 minutes on each side, or until the fish is opaque and flakes easily with a fork.
5. Remove from the grill and place on serving plates.
6. Garnish with lemon slices and fresh parsley.
7. Serve immediately.

Nutrition Info (per serving):
- Calories: 250
- Protein: 35g
- Carbohydrates: 2g
- Fat: 10g
- Fiber: 1g
- Sugar: 1g

Serves: 4
Cooking Time: 10 minutes

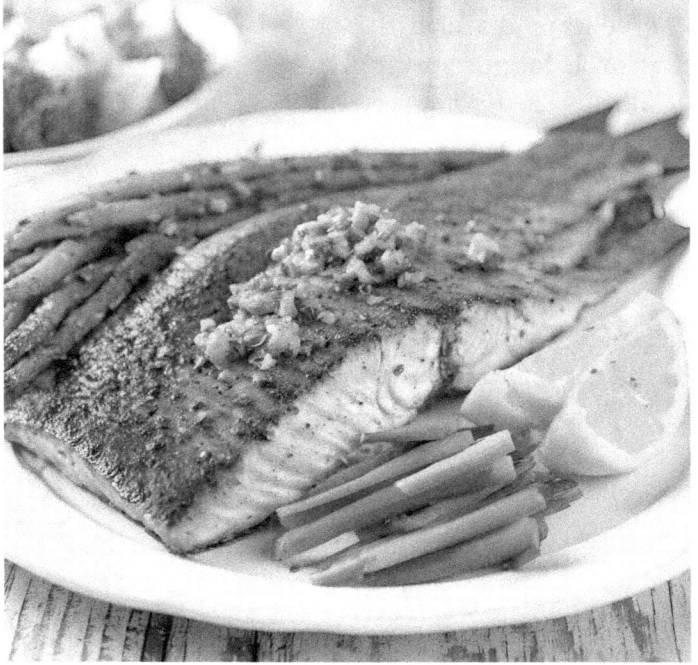

19. Clam Chowder with Skim Milk

Ingredients:
- 2 cups low-sodium vegetable broth
- 1 cup skim milk
- 2 tablespoons olive oil
- 1 onion, finely chopped
- 2 cloves garlic, minced
- 2 celery stalks, chopped
- 2 medium potatoes, peeled and diced
- 2 cups chopped clams (fresh or canned, drained)
- 1/2 teaspoon dried thyme
- 1/2 teaspoon ground black pepper
- 1/4 cup fresh parsley, chopped

Instructions:
1. In a large pot, heat the olive oil over medium heat. Add the onion, garlic, and celery, and sauté for 3-4 minutes until softened.
2. Add the diced potatoes and vegetable broth. Bring to a boil, then reduce heat and simmer for 15 minutes, or until the potatoes are tender.
3. Stir in the chopped clams, skim milk, dried thyme, and ground black pepper. Simmer for another 5-7 minutes, stirring occasionally.
4. Remove from heat and let cool slightly before serving.
5. Garnish with fresh parsley.
6. Serve immediately.

Nutrition Info (per serving):
- Calories: 200
- Protein: 15g
- Carbohydrates: 25g
- Fat: 6g
- Fiber: 3g
- Sugar: 6g

Serves: 4
Cooking Time: 30 minutes

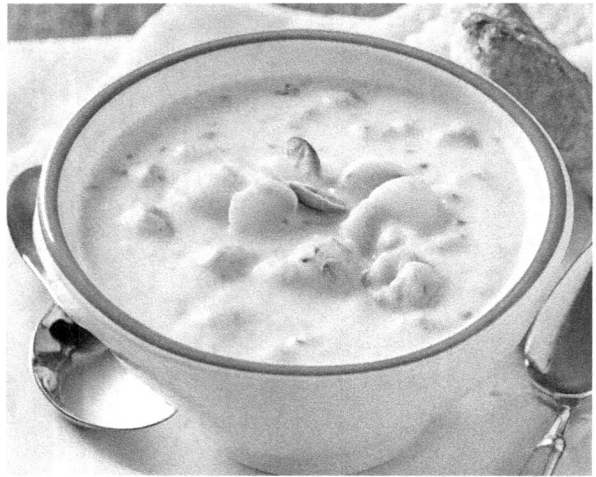

20. Basil Lime Scallops

Ingredients:
- 1 pound sea scallops
- 2 tablespoons olive oil
- 2 cloves garlic, minced
- 1 tablespoon fresh lime juice
- 1 tablespoon lime zest
- 1/4 cup fresh basil, chopped
- 1/2 teaspoon ground black pepper

Instructions:
1. Pat the scallops dry with a paper towel and season with ground black pepper.
2. Heat the olive oil in a large skillet over medium-high heat.
3. Add the minced garlic and sauté for 1-2 minutes until fragrant.
4. Add the scallops to the skillet and sear for 2-3 minutes on each side until golden brown and cooked through.
5. Remove the scallops from the skillet and place on a serving plate.
6. Drizzle with fresh lime juice and sprinkle with lime zest and fresh basil.
7. Serve immediately.

Nutrition Info (per serving):
- Calories: 220
- Protein: 25g
- Carbohydrates: 4g
- Fat: 10g
- Fiber: 1g
- Sugar: 1g

Serves: 4
Cooking Time: 10 minutes

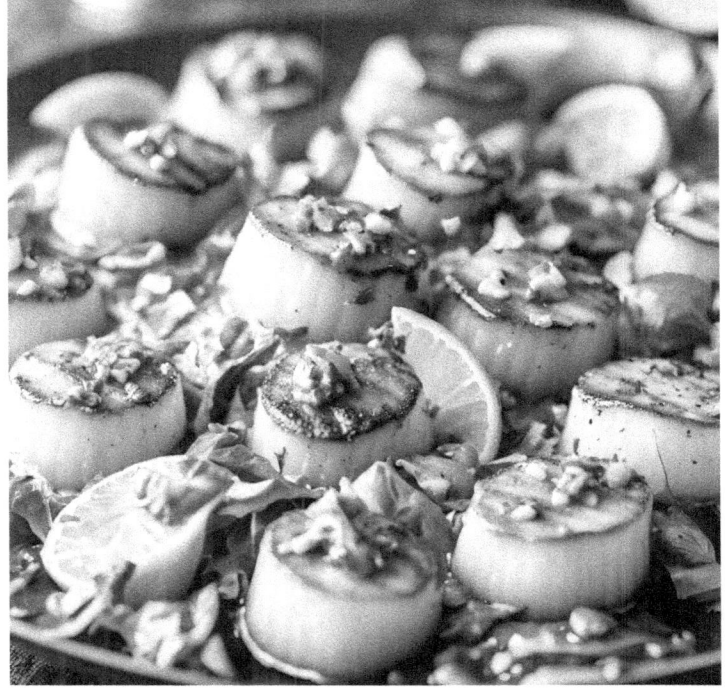

21. Turmeric-Ginger Marinated Halibut

Ingredients:
- 4 halibut fillets (about 6 ounces each)
- 1 tablespoon olive oil
- 1 tablespoon fresh ginger, grated
- 1 teaspoon ground turmeric
- 1 tablespoon fresh lemon juice
- 1/2 teaspoon ground black pepper
- 1/4 cup fresh cilantro, chopped

Instructions:
1. In a small bowl, whisk together the olive oil, fresh ginger, ground turmeric, lemon juice, and ground black pepper.
2. Place the halibut fillets in a shallow dish and pour the marinade over them. Cover and marinate in the refrigerator for at least 30 minutes.
3. Preheat the oven to 375°F (190°C).
4. Place the marinated halibut fillets on a baking sheet lined with parchment paper.
5. Bake for 15-20 minutes, or until the fish is opaque and flakes easily with a fork.
6. Garnish with fresh cilantro before serving.
7. Serve immediately.

Nutrition Info (per serving):
- Calories: 230
- Protein: 35g
- Carbohydrates: 2g
- Fat: 9g
- Fiber: 1g
- Sugar: 0g

Serves: 4
Cooking Time: 20 minutes (plus marinating time)

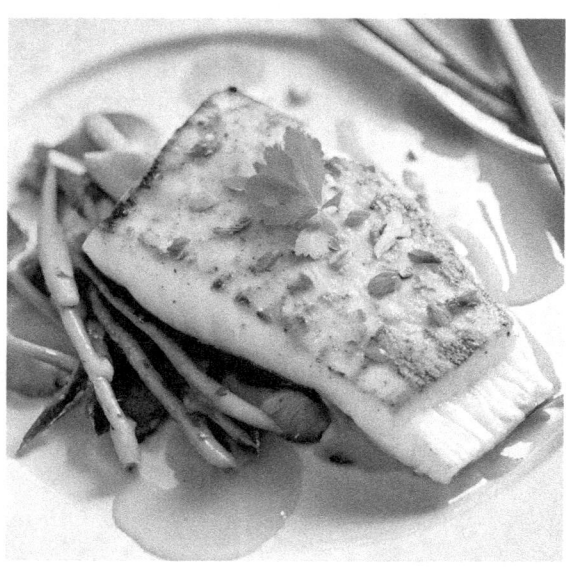

22. Fish Veracruz with Tomatoes and Olives

Ingredients:
- 4 white fish fillets (such as cod or snapper, about 6 ounces each)
- 2 tablespoons olive oil
- 1 onion, finely chopped
- 2 cloves garlic, minced
- 2 cups diced tomatoes (canned, no added salt)
- 1/4 cup green olives, sliced
- 1/4 cup black olives, sliced
- 1 tablespoon capers
- 1 tablespoon fresh lime juice
- 1/2 teaspoon dried oregano
- 1/2 teaspoon ground black pepper
- 1/4 cup fresh cilantro, chopped

Instructions:
1. Preheat the oven to 375°F (190°C).
2. In a large skillet, heat the olive oil over medium heat. Add the onion and garlic, and sauté for 2-3 minutes until softened.
3. Stir in the diced tomatoes, green olives, black olives, capers, lime juice, dried oregano, and ground black pepper. Simmer for 5 minutes.
4. Place the fish fillets in a baking dish and pour the tomato mixture over them.
5. Bake for 20-25 minutes, or until the fish is opaque and flakes easily with a fork.
6. Garnish with fresh cilantro before serving.
7. Serve immediately.

Nutrition Info (per serving):
- Calories: 250
- Protein: 35g
- Carbohydrates: 8g
- Fat: 9g
- Fiber: 3g
- Sugar: 4g

Serves: 4
Cooking Time: 25 minutes

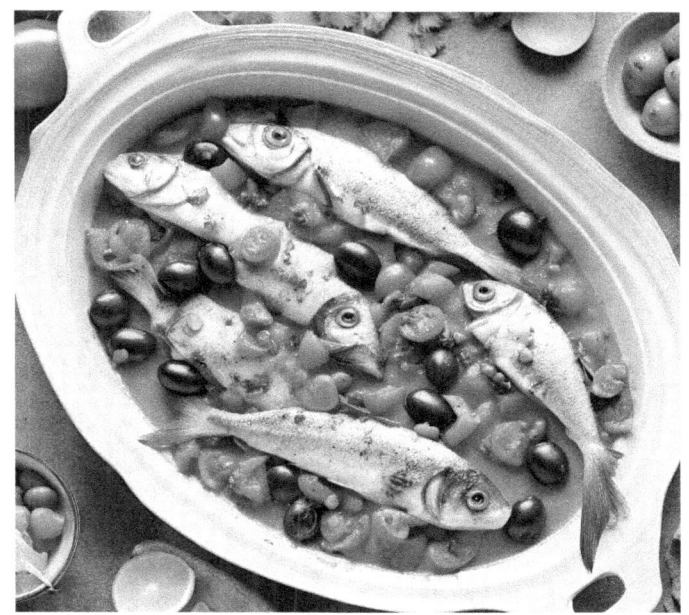

23. Sesame Ginger Tuna Steaks

Ingredients:
- 4 tuna steaks (about 6 ounces each)
- 2 tablespoons low-sodium soy sauce
- 1 tablespoon fresh ginger, grated
- 1 tablespoon sesame oil
- 1 tablespoon sesame seeds
- 1 tablespoon fresh lime juice
- 1/2 teaspoon ground black pepper
- 1/4 cup green onions, sliced

Instructions:
1. In a small bowl, whisk together the soy sauce, ginger, sesame oil, lime juice, and ground black pepper.
2. Place the tuna steaks in a shallow dish and pour the marinade over them. Cover and marinate in the refrigerator for at least 30 minutes.
3. Heat a non-stick skillet over medium-high heat.
4. Remove the tuna steaks from the marinade and sprinkle with sesame seeds.
5. Sear the tuna steaks for 2-3 minutes on each side, or until desired doneness.
6. Garnish with sliced green onions before serving.
7. Serve immediately.

Nutrition Info (per serving):
- Calories: 300
- Protein: 40g
- Carbohydrates: 3g
- Fat: 15g
- Fiber: 1g
- Sugar: 1g

Serves: 4
Cooking Time: 10 minutes (plus marinating time)

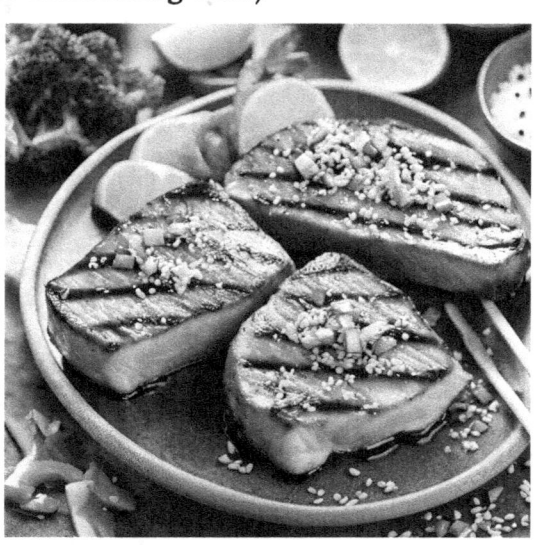

24. Steamed Blue Crabs

Ingredients:
- 4 large blue crabs, cleaned
- 2 cups water
- 1 cup apple cider vinegar
- 2 tablespoons Old Bay seasoning
- 2 cloves garlic, minced
- 1 lemon, cut into wedges
- 1/4 cup fresh parsley, chopped

Instructions:
1. In a large pot, combine the water, apple cider vinegar, Old Bay seasoning, and minced garlic. Bring to a boil.
2. Place a steamer basket in the pot.
3. Add the blue crabs to the steamer basket.
4. Cover and steam for 20-25 minutes, or until the crabs are bright red and cooked through.
5. Remove the crabs from the pot and place on a serving platter.
6. Garnish with lemon wedges and fresh parsley.
7. Serve immediately.

Nutrition Info (per serving):
- Calories: 200
- Protein: 30g
- Carbohydrates: 3g
- Fat: 6g
- Fiber: 1g
- Sugar: 1g

Serves: 4
Cooking Time: 25 minutes

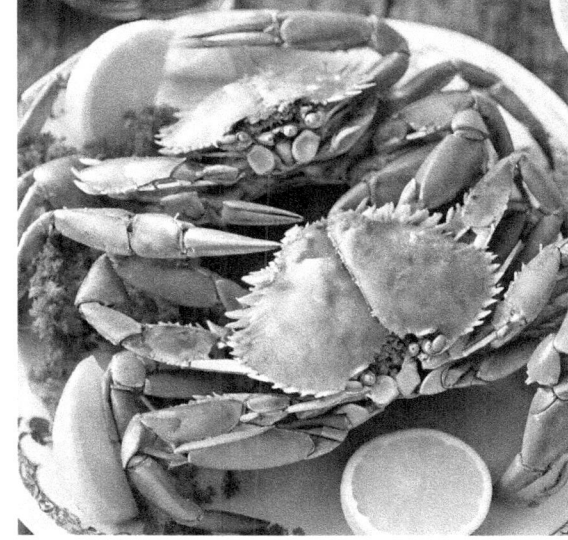

25. Paprika-Dusted Salmon

Ingredients:
- 4 salmon fillets (about 6 ounces each)
- 2 tablespoons olive oil
- 1 teaspoon smoked paprika
- 1/2 teaspoon garlic powder
- 1/2 teaspoon ground cumin
- 1/2 teaspoon ground black pepper
- 1 lemon, cut into wedges

Instructions:
1. Preheat the oven to 375°F (190°C).
2. In a small bowl, combine the olive oil, smoked paprika, garlic powder, ground cumin, and ground black pepper.
3. Brush both sides of the salmon fillets with the olive oil mixture.
4. Place the salmon fillets on a baking sheet lined with parchment paper.
5. Bake for 15-20 minutes, or until the salmon is cooked through and flakes easily with a fork.
6. Garnish with lemon wedges before serving.
7. Serve immediately.

Nutrition Info (per serving):
- Calories: 320
- Protein: 32g
- Carbohydrates: 2g
- Fat: 20g
- Fiber: 1g
- Sugar: 0g

Serves: 4
Cooking Time: 20 minutes

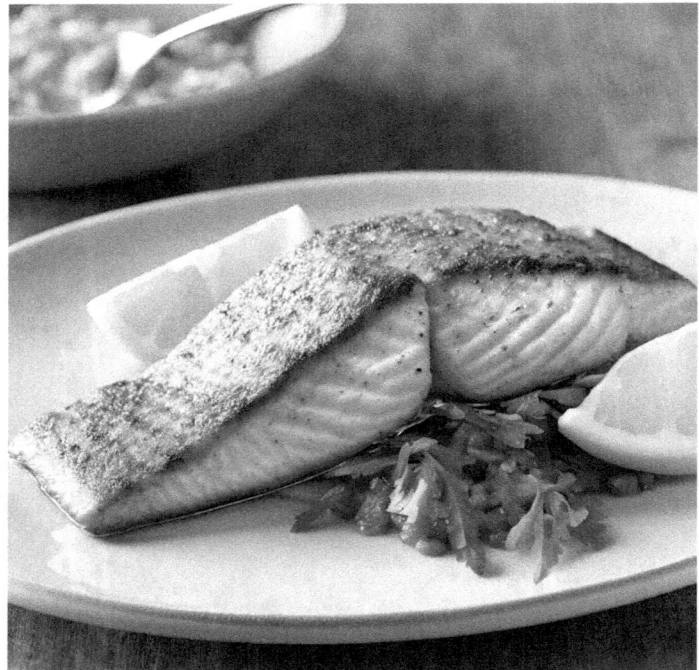

Poultry Recipes

1. Turkey and Mushroom Pilaf
Ingredients:
- 1 cup brown rice
- 2 cups low-sodium chicken broth
- 1 tablespoon olive oil
- 1 pound ground turkey
- 1 onion, finely chopped
- 2 cloves garlic, minced
- 2 cups mushrooms, sliced
- 1/2 teaspoon dried thyme
- 1/2 teaspoon ground black pepper
- 1/4 cup fresh parsley, chopped

Instructions:
1. In a medium saucepan, bring the chicken broth to a boil. Add the brown rice, reduce heat to low, cover, and simmer for 40 minutes or until the rice is tender and the liquid is absorbed.
2. While the rice is cooking, heat the olive oil in a large skillet over medium heat. Add the ground turkey, onion, and garlic, and cook until the turkey is browned and the onion is softened, about 5-7 minutes.
3. Add the mushrooms, dried thyme, and ground black pepper to the skillet. Cook for an additional 5 minutes, stirring occasionally, until the mushrooms are tender.
4. Stir the cooked rice into the turkey and mushroom mixture until well combined.
5. Remove from heat and sprinkle with fresh parsley before serving.
6. Serve immediately.

Nutrition Info (per serving):
- Calories: 320
- Protein: 28g
- Carbohydrates: 36g
- Fat: 10g
- Fiber: 4g
- Sugar: 3g

Serves: 4
Cooking Time: 50 minutes

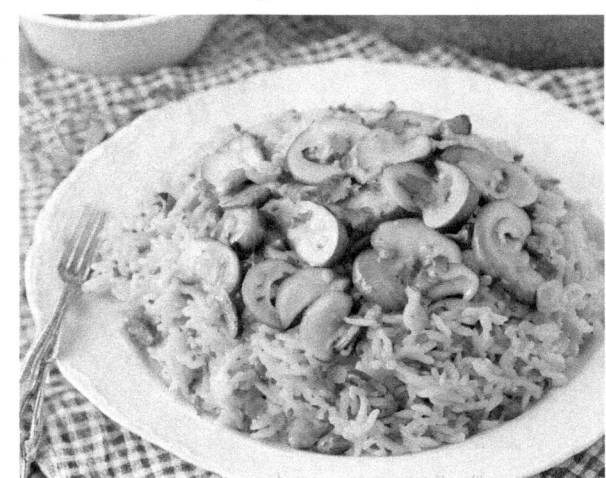

2. Balsamic Glazed Chicken Breasts

Ingredients:
- 4 boneless, skinless chicken breasts (about 6 ounces each)
- 2 tablespoons olive oil
- 1/4 cup balsamic vinegar
- 2 cloves garlic, minced
- 1 tablespoon honey
- 1/2 teaspoon dried oregano
- 1/2 teaspoon ground black pepper
- 1/4 cup fresh basil, chopped

Instructions:
1. Preheat the oven to 375°F (190°C).
2. In a small bowl, whisk together the olive oil, balsamic vinegar, minced garlic, honey, dried oregano, and ground black pepper.
3. Place the chicken breasts in a baking dish and pour the balsamic mixture over them, turning to coat both sides.
4. Bake for 25-30 minutes, or until the chicken is cooked through and the internal temperature reaches 165°F (74°C).
5. Remove from the oven and let rest for 5 minutes.
6. Garnish with fresh basil before serving.
7. Serve immediately.

Nutrition Info (per serving):
- Calories: 280
- Protein: 36g
- Carbohydrates: 8g
- Fat: 10g
- Fiber: 1g
- Sugar: 6g

Serves: 4
Cooking Time: 30 minutes

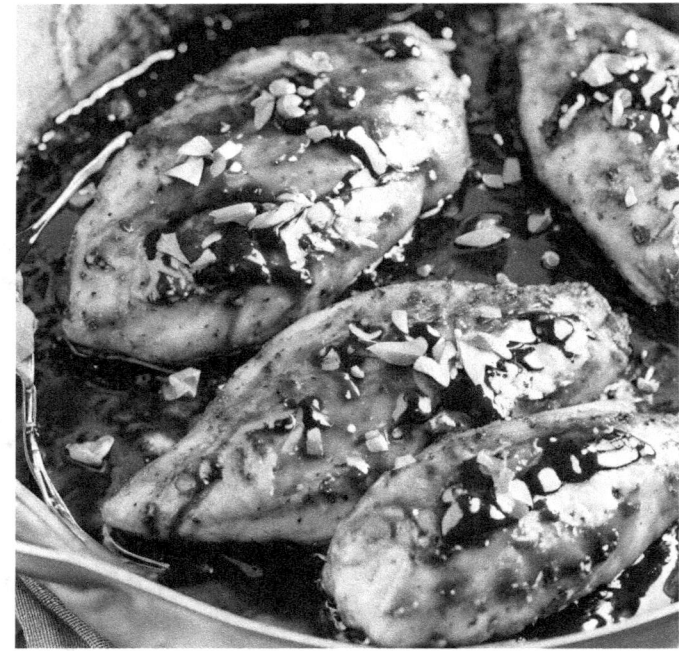

3. Lime and Cilantro Turkey Patties

Ingredients:
- 1 pound ground turkey
- 1/4 cup breadcrumbs (whole wheat or gluten-free)
- 1 egg, lightly beaten
- 2 tablespoons fresh lime juice
- 1 tablespoon lime zest
- 1/4 cup fresh cilantro, chopped
- 2 cloves garlic, minced
- 1/2 teaspoon ground cumin
- 1/2 teaspoon ground black pepper
- 1 tablespoon olive oil

Instructions:
1. In a large bowl, combine the ground turkey, breadcrumbs, egg, lime juice, lime zest, cilantro, garlic, ground cumin, and ground black pepper. Mix until well combined.
2. Form the mixture into 8 patties.
3. Heat the olive oil in a large skillet over medium heat.
4. Add the patties to the skillet and cook for 4-5 minutes on each side, or until the patties are cooked through and the internal temperature reaches 165°F (74°C).
5. Remove from the skillet and let rest for a few minutes before serving.
6. Serve immediately.

Nutrition Info (per serving):
- Calories: 210
- Protein: 20g
- Carbohydrates: 5g
- Fat: 12g
- Fiber: 1g
- Sugar: 1g

Serves: 4
Cooking Time: 20 minutes

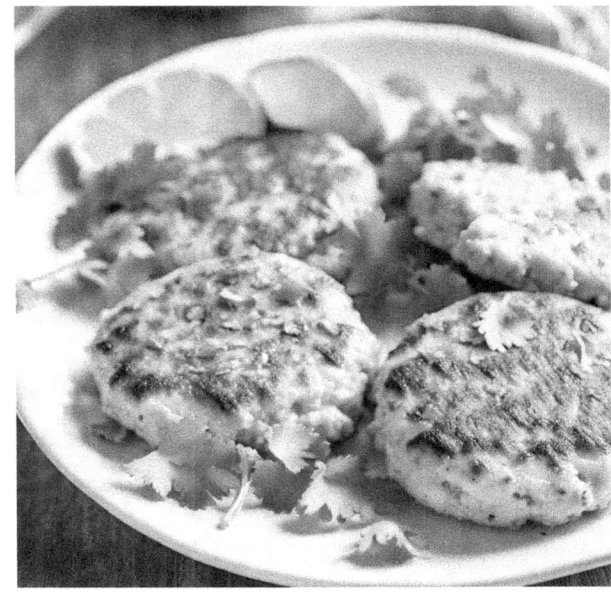

4. Salsa Fresca Chicken Bake

Ingredients:
- 4 boneless, skinless chicken breasts (about 6 ounces each)
- 1 cup fresh tomato salsa (homemade or store-bought, no added sugars)
- 1/2 cup shredded low-fat mozzarella cheese
- 1/4 cup fresh cilantro, chopped
- 1 tablespoon olive oil
- 1 teaspoon ground cumin
- 1/2 teaspoon ground black pepper

Instructions:
1. Preheat the oven to 375°F (190°C).
2. In a small bowl, mix together the olive oil, ground cumin, and ground black pepper.
3. Brush the chicken breasts with the olive oil mixture and place them in a baking dish.
4. Spread the fresh tomato salsa evenly over the chicken breasts.
5. Sprinkle the shredded mozzarella cheese over the salsa.
6. Bake for 25-30 minutes, or until the chicken is cooked through and the internal temperature reaches 165°F (74°C).
7. Remove from the oven and let rest for 5 minutes.
8. Garnish with fresh cilantro before serving.
9. Serve immediately.

Nutrition Info (per serving):
- Calories: 280
- Protein: 36g
- Carbohydrates: 6g
- Fat: 12g
- Fiber: 2g
- Sugar: 3g

Serves: 4
Cooking Time: 30 minutes

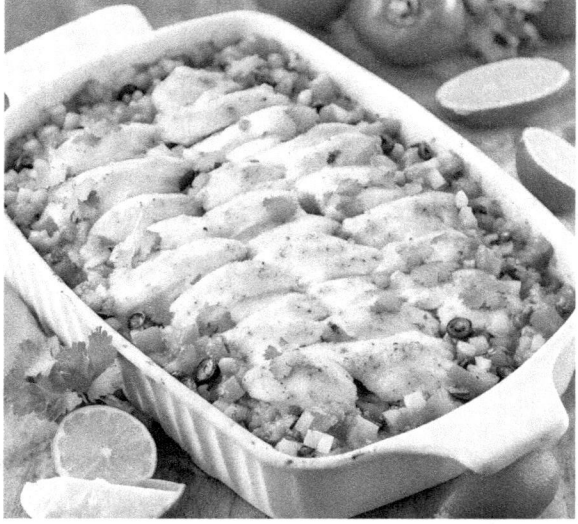

5. Chicken Ratatouille

Ingredients:
- 4 boneless, skinless chicken breasts (about 6 ounces each)
- 1 tablespoon olive oil
- 1 onion, chopped
- 2 cloves garlic, minced
- 1 eggplant, diced
- 2 zucchinis, sliced
- 1 red bell pepper, chopped
- 1 yellow bell pepper, chopped
- 2 cups diced tomatoes (canned, no added salt)
- 1 teaspoon dried thyme
- 1 teaspoon dried basil
- 1/2 teaspoon ground black pepper
- 1/4 cup fresh parsley, chopped

Instructions:
1. Preheat the oven to 375°F (190°C).
2. In a large skillet, heat the olive oil over medium heat. Add the onion and garlic, and sauté for 3-4 minutes until softened.
3. Add the diced eggplant, zucchinis, red bell pepper, and yellow bell pepper. Cook for another 5 minutes, stirring occasionally.
4. Stir in the diced tomatoes, dried thyme, dried basil, and ground black pepper. Simmer for 10 minutes.
5. Place the chicken breasts in a baking dish and pour the vegetable mixture over the top.
6. Cover the baking dish with aluminum foil and bake for 25-30 minutes, or until the chicken is cooked through and the internal temperature reaches 165°F (74°C).
7. Remove from the oven and let rest for 5 minutes.
8. Garnish with fresh parsley before serving.
9. Serve immediately.

Nutrition Info (per serving):
- Calories: 320
- Protein: 36g
- Carbohydrates: 18g
- Fat: 12g
- Fiber: 6g
- Sugar: 10g

Serves: 4
Cooking Time: 40 minutes

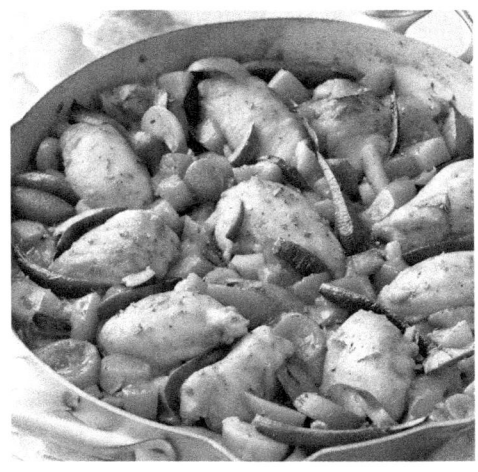

6. Herb Roasted Turkey Thighs

Ingredients:
- 4 turkey thighs (about 8 ounces each)
- 2 tablespoons olive oil
- 1 tablespoon fresh rosemary, chopped
- 1 tablespoon fresh thyme, chopped
- 2 cloves garlic, minced
- 1/2 teaspoon ground black pepper
- 1 lemon, thinly sliced

Instructions:
1. Preheat the oven to 375°F (190°C).
2. In a small bowl, mix together the olive oil, rosemary, thyme, garlic, and ground black pepper.
3. Rub the olive oil mixture all over the turkey thighs.
4. Place the turkey thighs in a roasting pan and top with lemon slices.
5. Roast for 45-50 minutes, or until the internal temperature reaches 165°F (74°C).
6. Remove from the oven and let rest for 10 minutes.
7. Serve immediately.

Nutrition Info (per serving):
- Calories: 350
- Protein: 38g
- Carbohydrates: 2g
- Fat: 20g
- Fiber: 1g
- Sugar: 1g

Serves: 4
Cooking Time: 50 minutes

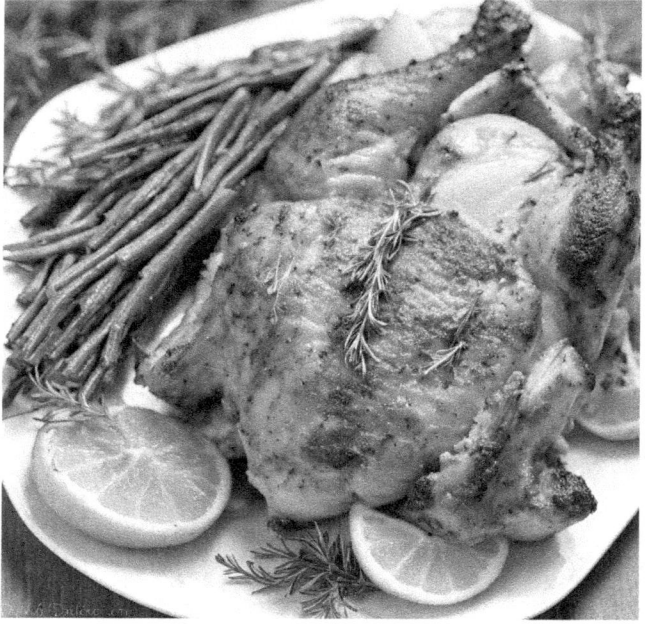

7. Chicken Piccata without Capers

Ingredients:
- 4 boneless, skinless chicken breasts (about 6 ounces each)
- 1/4 cup whole wheat flour
- 2 tablespoons olive oil
- 1/2 cup low-sodium chicken broth
- 1/4 cup fresh lemon juice
- 2 cloves garlic, minced
- 1/2 teaspoon dried oregano
- 1/2 teaspoon ground black pepper
- 1/4 cup fresh parsley, chopped

Instructions:
1. Lightly coat the chicken breasts with whole wheat flour.
2. In a large skillet, heat the olive oil over medium heat. Add the chicken breasts and cook for 3-4 minutes on each side, or until golden brown and cooked through. Remove from the skillet and set aside.
3. In the same skillet, add the chicken broth, lemon juice, garlic, dried oregano, and ground black pepper. Bring to a simmer and cook for 2-3 minutes.
4. Return the chicken breasts to the skillet and cook for another 2 minutes, coating them with the sauce.
5. Remove from heat and sprinkle with fresh parsley before serving.
6. Serve immediately.

Nutrition Info (per serving):
- Calories: 280
- Protein: 36g
- Carbohydrates: 6g
- Fat: 12g
- Fiber: 1g
- Sugar: 1g

Serves: 4
Cooking Time: 20 minutes

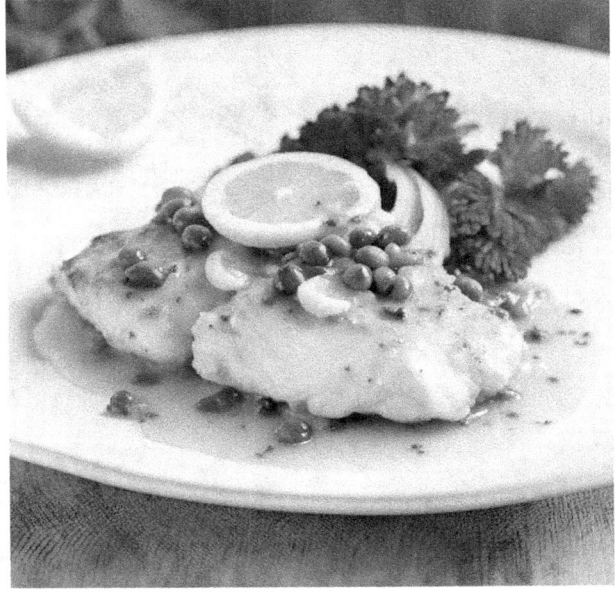

8. Grilled Turkey Breast with Cranberry Glaze

Ingredients:
- 4 turkey breast cutlets (about 6 ounces each)
- 2 tablespoons olive oil
- 1/2 cup cranberry juice (no added sugar)
- 1/4 cup fresh cranberries (or dried, unsweetened)
- 1 tablespoon honey
- 1 tablespoon balsamic vinegar
- 1/2 teaspoon ground black pepper
- 1/4 cup fresh thyme, chopped

Instructions:
1. In a small saucepan, combine the cranberry juice, fresh cranberries, honey, balsamic vinegar, and ground black pepper. Bring to a boil, then reduce heat and simmer for 10 minutes until the cranberries have softened and the mixture has thickened.
2. Preheat the grill to medium-high heat.
3. Brush the turkey breast cutlets with olive oil.
4. Grill the turkey cutlets for 4-5 minutes on each side, or until the internal temperature reaches 165°F (74°C).
5. Brush the cranberry glaze over the turkey cutlets during the last minute of grilling.
6. Remove from the grill and let rest for a few minutes.
7. Garnish with fresh thyme before serving.
8. Serve immediately.

Nutrition Info (per serving):
- Calories: 290
- Protein: 36g
- Carbohydrates: 10g
- Fat: 12g
- Fiber: 1g
- Sugar: 8g

Serves: 4
Cooking Time: 20 minutes

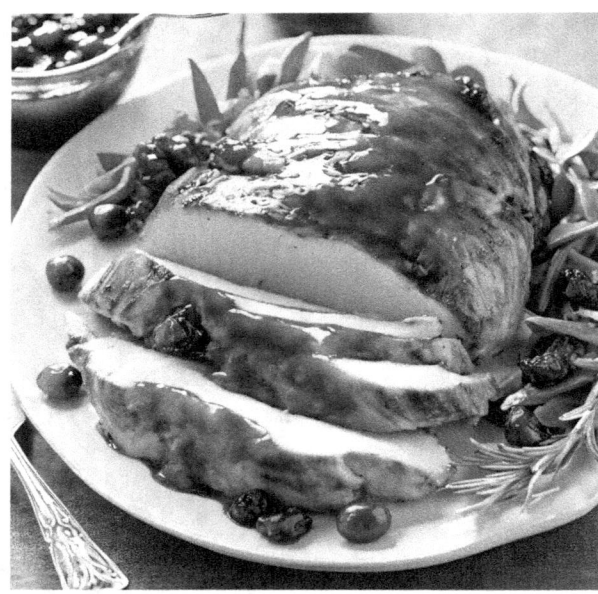

9. Chicken Cacciatore with Mushrooms

Ingredients:
- 4 boneless, skinless chicken thighs (about 6 ounces each)
- 2 tablespoons olive oil
- 1 onion, chopped
- 2 cloves garlic, minced
- 2 cups mushrooms, sliced
- 1 red bell pepper, chopped
- 1 cup low-sodium chicken broth
- 1 cup diced tomatoes (canned, no added salt)
- 1 teaspoon dried basil
- 1/2 teaspoon ground black pepper
- 1/4 cup fresh basil, chopped

Instructions:
1. In a large skillet, heat the olive oil over medium heat. Add the chicken thighs and cook for 4-5 minutes on each side until browned. Remove from the skillet and set aside.
2. In the same skillet, add the onion and garlic. Sauté for 2-3 minutes until softened.
3. Add the mushrooms and red bell pepper, and cook for another 5 minutes.
4. Stir in the chicken broth, diced tomatoes, dried basil, and ground black pepper. Bring to a simmer.
5. Return the chicken thighs to the skillet and cook for 20 minutes, or until the chicken is cooked through and tender.
6. Remove from heat and let rest for a few minutes.
7. Garnish with fresh basil before serving.
8. Serve immediately.

Nutrition Info (per serving):
- Calories: 320
- Protein: 30g
- Carbohydrates: 10g
- Fat: 18g
- Fiber: 3g
- Sugar: 6g

Serves: 4
Cooking Time: 30 minutes

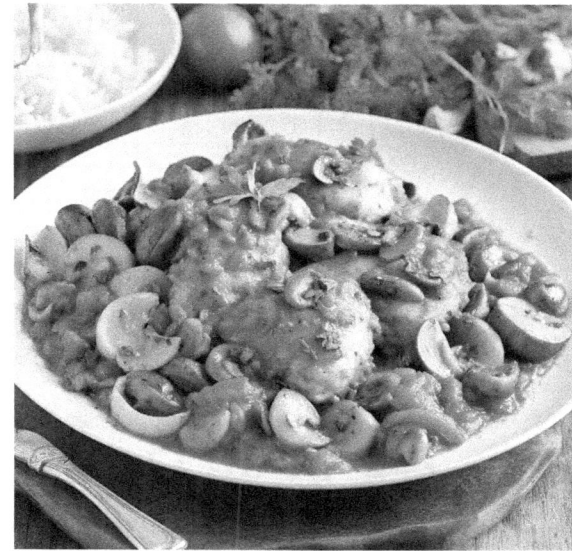

10. Orange Rosemary Chicken

Ingredients:
- 4 boneless, skinless chicken breasts (about 6 ounces each)
- 1/4 cup fresh orange juice
- 1 tablespoon orange zest
- 2 tablespoons olive oil
- 2 cloves garlic, minced
- 1 tablespoon fresh rosemary, chopped
- 1/2 teaspoon ground black pepper

Instructions:
1. Preheat the oven to 375°F (190°C).
2. In a small bowl, whisk together the orange juice, orange zest, olive oil, garlic, rosemary, and ground black pepper.
3. Place the chicken breasts in a baking dish and pour the orange mixture over them, turning to coat both sides.
4. Bake for 25-30 minutes, or until the chicken is cooked through and the internal temperature reaches 165°F (74°C).
5. Remove from the oven and let rest for 5 minutes before serving.
6. Serve immediately.

Nutrition Info (per serving):
- Calories: 250
- Protein: 36g
- Carbohydrates: 4g
- Fat: 10g
- Fiber: 1g
- Sugar: 3g

Serves: 4
Cooking Time: 30 minutes

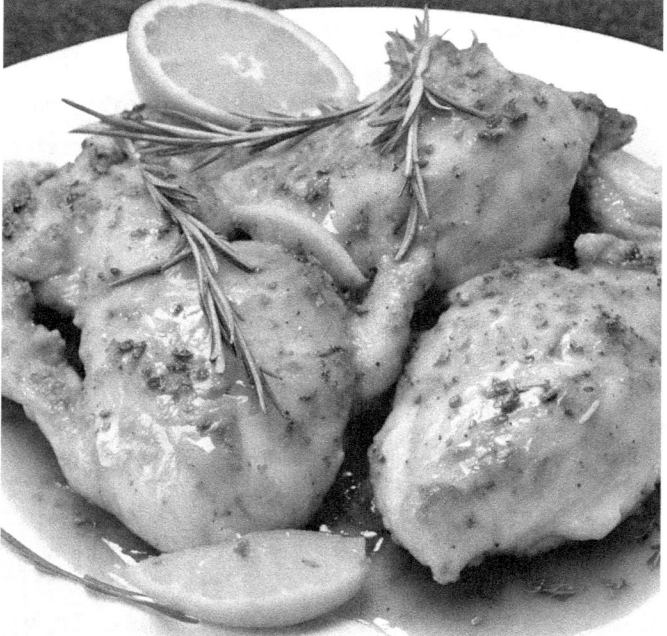

11. Turkey Taco Soup

Ingredients:
- 1 pound ground turkey
- 1 tablespoon olive oil
- 1 onion, chopped
- 2 cloves garlic, minced
- 1 red bell pepper, chopped
- 1 green bell pepper, chopped
- 1 cup frozen corn
- 1 can (15 ounces) black beans, rinsed and drained
- 1 can (15 ounces) diced tomatoes (no added salt)
- 4 cups low-sodium chicken broth
- 1 tablespoon chili powder
- 1 teaspoon ground cumin
- 1/2 teaspoon ground black pepper
- 1/4 cup fresh cilantro, chopped

Instructions:
1. In a large pot, heat the olive oil over medium heat. Add the ground turkey and cook until browned, about 5-7 minutes.
2. Add the onion and garlic, and sauté for 2-3 minutes until softened.
3. Stir in the red bell pepper, green bell pepper, corn, black beans, diced tomatoes, chicken broth, chili powder, ground cumin, and ground black pepper.
4. Bring to a boil, then reduce heat and simmer for 20 minutes.
5. Remove from heat and let cool slightly before serving.
6. Garnish with fresh cilantro.
7. Serve immediately.

Nutrition Info (per serving):
- Calories: 280
- Protein: 25g
- Carbohydrates: 28g
- Fat: 10g
- Fiber: 8g
- Sugar: 6g

Serves: 6
Cooking Time: 30 minutes

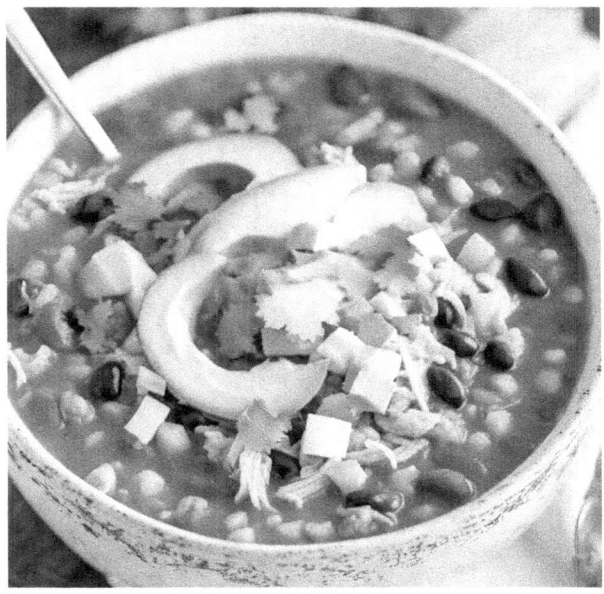

12. Chicken and Asparagus Stir Fry

Ingredients:
- 1 pound boneless, skinless chicken breast, cut into thin strips
- 1 tablespoon olive oil
- 2 cloves garlic, minced
- 1 tablespoon fresh ginger, grated
- 1 bunch asparagus, cut into 2-inch pieces
- 1 red bell pepper, sliced
- 1/4 cup low-sodium soy sauce
- 2 tablespoons fresh lime juice
- 1 tablespoon honey
- 1/2 teaspoon ground black pepper

Instructions:
1. In a small bowl, whisk together the soy sauce, lime juice, honey, and ground black pepper. Set aside.
2. Heat the olive oil in a large skillet or wok over medium-high heat.
3. Add the chicken strips and cook for 4-5 minutes until browned and cooked through. Remove from the skillet and set aside.
4. In the same skillet, add the garlic and ginger, and sauté for 1-2 minutes until fragrant.
5. Add the asparagus and red bell pepper, and stir-fry for 3-4 minutes until tender-crisp.
6. Return the chicken to the skillet and pour the soy sauce mixture over the top. Stir to coat and cook for another 2 minutes.
7. Remove from heat and serve immediately.

Nutrition Info (per serving):
- Calories: 240
- Protein: 30g
- Carbohydrates: 12g
- Fat: 8g
- Fiber: 4g
- Sugar: 6g

Serves: 4
Cooking Time: 20 minutes

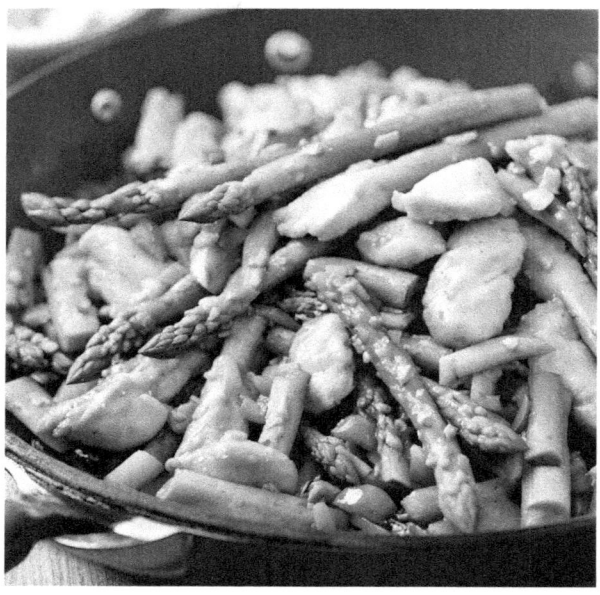

13. Chicken and Broccoli Alfredo

Ingredients:
- 1 pound boneless, skinless chicken breast, cut into bite-sized pieces
- 2 cups broccoli florets
- 1 tablespoon olive oil
- 2 cloves garlic, minced
- 1 cup low-fat milk
- 1/2 cup low-fat Parmesan cheese, grated
- 1 tablespoon whole wheat flour
- 1/2 teaspoon ground black pepper
- 1/4 teaspoon ground nutmeg
- 8 ounces whole wheat fettuccine, cooked according to package instructions

Instructions:
1. In a large skillet, heat the olive oil over medium heat. Add the chicken pieces and cook for 5-7 minutes until browned and cooked through. Remove from the skillet and set aside.
2. In the same skillet, add the garlic and sauté for 1-2 minutes until fragrant.
3. Add the whole wheat flour and cook, stirring constantly, for 1 minute.
4. Gradually whisk in the low-fat milk and bring to a simmer. Cook for 3-4 minutes until thickened.
5. Stir in the grated Parmesan cheese, ground black pepper, and ground nutmeg. Cook for another 2 minutes until the cheese is melted and the sauce is smooth.
6. Return the chicken to the skillet and add the broccoli florets. Cook for 3-4 minutes until the broccoli is tender.
7. Toss the cooked fettuccine with the chicken and broccoli Alfredo sauce.
8. Serve immediately.

Nutrition Info (per serving):
- Calories: 350
- Protein: 30g
- Carbohydrates: 42g
- Fat: 10g
- Fiber: 6g
- Sugar: 6g

Serves: 4
Cooking Time: 30 minutes

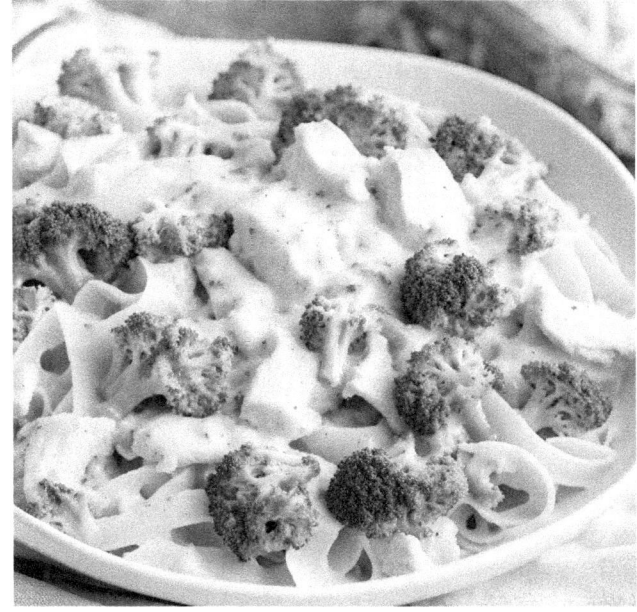

14. Baked Turkey Cutlets with Sage

Ingredients:
- 4 turkey cutlets (about 6 ounces each)
- 2 tablespoons olive oil
- 1 tablespoon fresh sage, chopped
- 2 cloves garlic, minced
- 1/2 teaspoon ground black pepper
- 1/4 cup low-sodium chicken broth
- 1 tablespoon fresh lemon juice

Instructions:
1. Preheat the oven to 375°F (190°C).
2. In a small bowl, mix together the olive oil, sage, garlic, and ground black pepper.
3. Rub the olive oil mixture all over the turkey cutlets.
4. Place the turkey cutlets in a baking dish and pour the chicken broth and lemon juice over them.
5. Bake for 20-25 minutes, or until the turkey is cooked through and the internal temperature reaches 165°F (74°C).
6. Remove from the oven and let rest for 5 minutes before serving.
7. Serve immediately.

Nutrition Info (per serving):
- Calories: 250
- Protein: 34g
- Carbohydrates: 2g
- Fat: 10g
- Fiber: 1g
- Sugar: 1g

Serves: 4
Cooking Time: 25 minutes

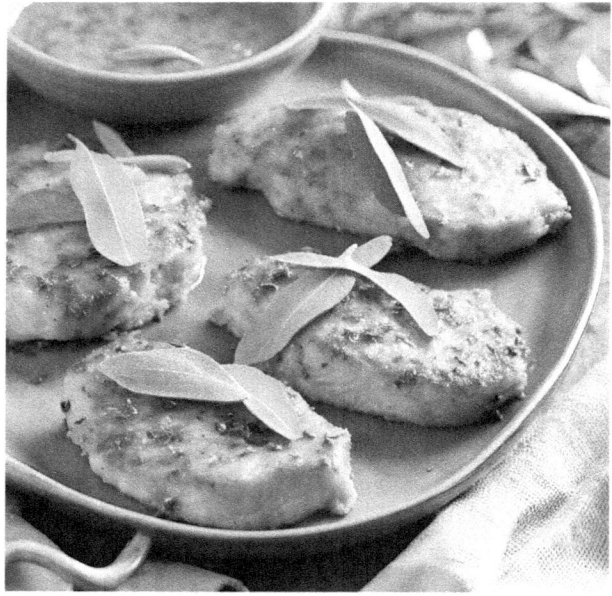

15. Chicken Soup with Barley

Ingredients:
- 1 pound boneless, skinless chicken breasts, diced
- 1 tablespoon olive oil
- 1 onion, chopped
- 2 cloves garlic, minced
- 3 carrots, sliced
- 3 celery stalks, sliced
- 1 cup pearl barley
- 6 cups low-sodium chicken broth
- 1 teaspoon dried thyme
- 1/2 teaspoon ground black pepper
- 1/4 cup fresh parsley, chopped

Instructions:
1. In a large pot, heat the olive oil over medium heat. Add the onion and garlic, and sauté for 3-4 minutes until softened.
2. Add the diced chicken and cook until browned, about 5-7 minutes.
3. Add the carrots, celery, pearl barley, chicken broth, dried thyme, and ground black pepper. Bring to a boil.
4. Reduce heat and simmer for 45-50 minutes, or until the barley is tender.
5. Remove from heat and stir in the fresh parsley.
6. Serve immediately.

Nutrition Info (per serving):
- Calories: 320
- Protein: 30g
- Carbohydrates: 35g
- Fat: 8g
- Fiber: 7g
- Sugar: 5g

Serves: 6
Cooking Time: 60 minutes

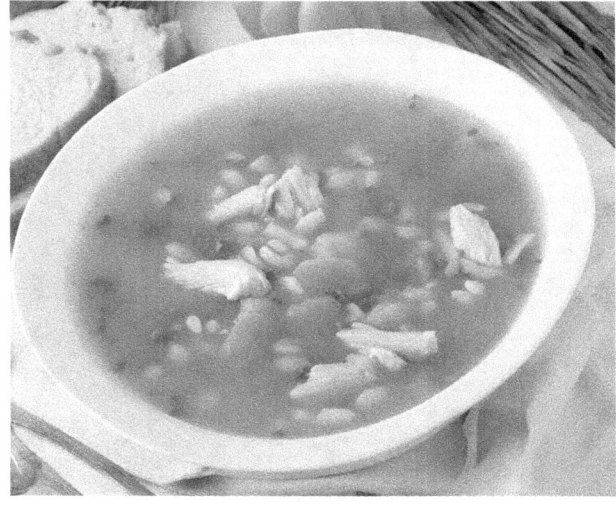

16. Lemon Garlic Roast Turkey

Ingredients:
- 1 turkey breast (about 2 pounds)
- 2 tablespoons olive oil
- 2 cloves garlic, minced
- 1 lemon, zested and juiced
- 1 tablespoon fresh rosemary, chopped
- 1/2 teaspoon ground black pepper

Instructions:
1. Preheat the oven to 375°F (190°C).
2. In a small bowl, mix together the olive oil, garlic, lemon zest, lemon juice, rosemary, and ground black pepper.
3. Rub the mixture all over the turkey breast.
4. Place the turkey breast in a roasting pan.
5. Roast for 60-70 minutes, or until the internal temperature reaches 165°F (74°C).
6. Remove from the oven and let rest for 10 minutes before slicing.
7. Serve immediately.

Nutrition Info (per serving):
- Calories: 240
- Protein: 36g
- Carbohydrates: 2g
- Fat: 9g
- Fiber: 1g
- Sugar: 1g

Serves: 6
Cooking Time: 70 minutes

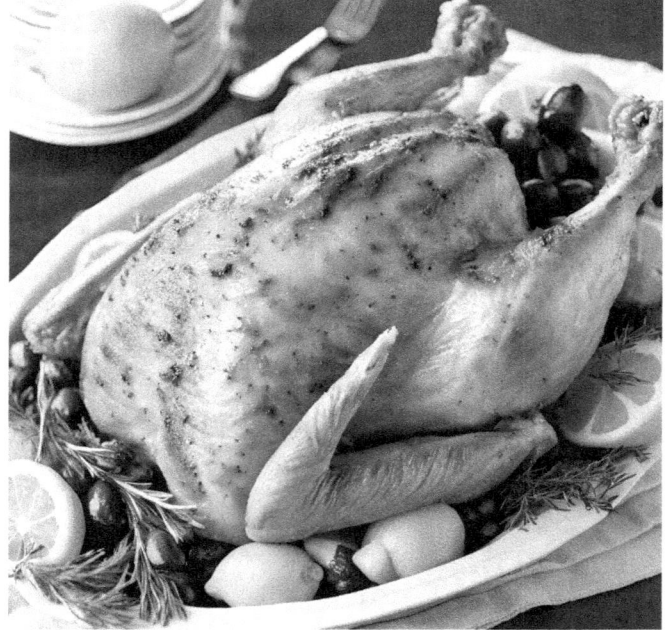

17. Turkey Spinach Meatloaf

Ingredients:
- 1 pound ground turkey
- 1 cup fresh spinach, chopped
- 1/2 cup whole wheat breadcrumbs
- 1/4 cup grated carrots
- 1 egg, lightly beaten
- 2 cloves garlic, minced
- 1 tablespoon fresh thyme, chopped
- 1/2 teaspoon ground black pepper

Instructions:
1. Preheat the oven to 375°F (190°C).
2. In a large bowl, combine the ground turkey, spinach, breadcrumbs, grated carrots, egg, garlic, thyme, and ground black pepper. Mix until well combined.
3. Shape the mixture into a loaf and place in a baking dish.
4. Bake for 45-50 minutes, or until the internal temperature reaches 165°F (74°C).
5. Remove from the oven and let rest for 5 minutes before slicing.
6. Serve immediately.

Nutrition Info (per serving):
- Calories: 220
- Protein: 28g
- Carbohydrates: 10g
- Fat: 8g
- Fiber: 2g
- Sugar: 2g

Serves: 4
Cooking Time: 50 minutes

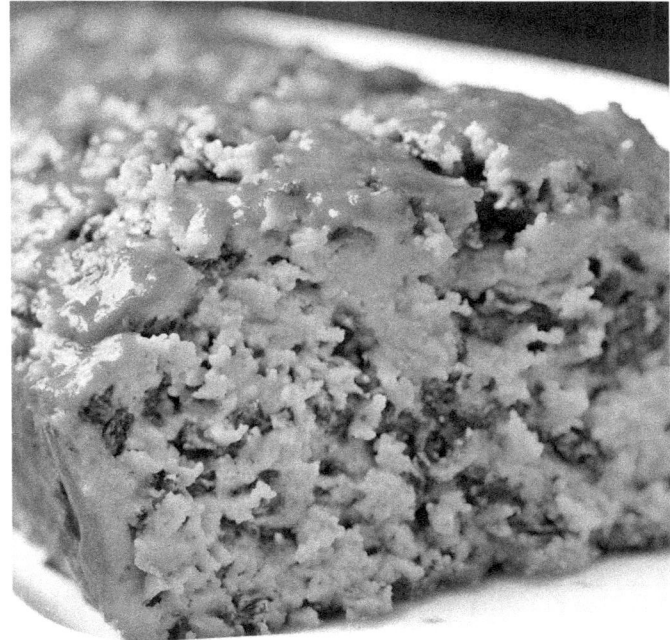

18. Chicken and Vegetable Kebabs

Ingredients:
- 1 pound boneless, skinless chicken breast, cut into 1-inch cubes
- 1 red bell pepper, cut into 1-inch pieces
- 1 yellow bell pepper, cut into 1-inch pieces
- 1 zucchini, sliced into rounds
- 1 red onion, cut into wedges
- 2 tablespoons olive oil
- 2 cloves garlic, minced
- 1 tablespoon fresh lemon juice
- 1 teaspoon dried oregano
- 1/2 teaspoon ground black pepper

Instructions:
1. In a large bowl, combine the olive oil, garlic, lemon juice, oregano, and ground black pepper.
2. Add the chicken and vegetables to the bowl and toss to coat.
3. Thread the chicken and vegetables onto skewers.
4. Preheat the grill to medium-high heat.
5. Grill the kebabs for 10-12 minutes, turning occasionally, until the chicken is cooked through and the vegetables are tender.
6. Serve immediately.

Nutrition Info (per serving):
- Calories: 240
- Protein: 28g
- Carbohydrates: 8g
- Fat: 10g
- Fiber: 3g
- Sugar: 5g

Serves: 4
Cooking Time: 20 minutes

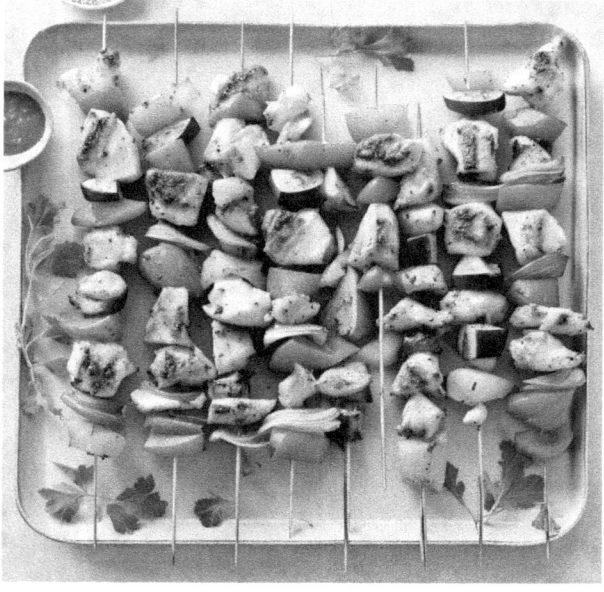

19. Turkey and Quinoa Stuffed Tomatoes

Ingredients:
- 4 large tomatoes
- 1/2 cup quinoa, rinsed
- 1 cup low-sodium chicken broth
- 1/2 pound ground turkey
- 1 tablespoon olive oil
- 1 onion, finely chopped
- 2 cloves garlic, minced
- 1 tablespoon fresh basil, chopped
- 1/2 teaspoon ground black pepper
- 1/4 cup grated low-fat mozzarella cheese

Instructions:
1. Preheat the oven to 375°F (190°C).
2. Slice the tops off the tomatoes and scoop out the insides, leaving a hollow shell. Set aside.
3. In a medium saucepan, bring the chicken broth to a boil. Add the quinoa, reduce heat to low, cover, and simmer for 15 minutes or until the quinoa is tender and the liquid is absorbed.
4. In a large skillet, heat the olive oil over medium heat. Add the onion and garlic, and sauté for 3-4 minutes until softened.
5. Add the ground turkey and cook until browned, about 5-7 minutes.
6. Stir in the cooked quinoa, basil, and ground black pepper. Cook for another 2 minutes.
7. Stuff the quinoa and turkey mixture into the hollowed tomatoes.
8. Place the stuffed tomatoes in a baking dish and top with grated mozzarella cheese.
9. Bake for 20 minutes, or until the cheese is melted and the tomatoes are tender.
10. Serve immediately.

Nutrition Info (per serving):
- Calories: 280
- Protein: 22g
- Carbohydrates: 22g
- Fat: 12g
- Fiber: 5g
- Sugar: 8g

Serves: 4
Cooking Time: 45 minutes

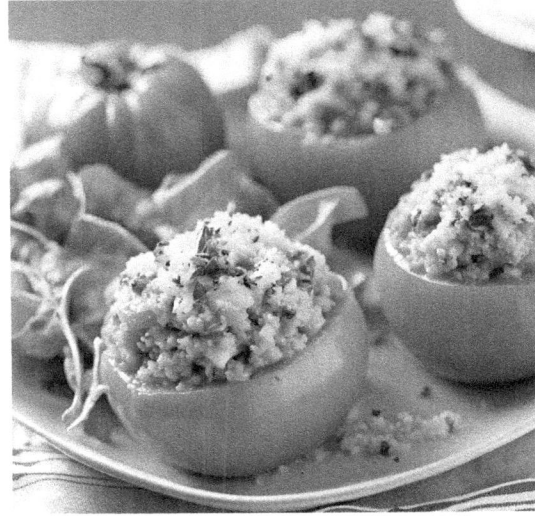

20. Asian Chicken Lettuce Cups

Ingredients:
- 1 pound ground chicken
- 2 tablespoons olive oil
- 2 cloves garlic, minced
- 1 tablespoon fresh ginger, grated
- 1/4 cup low-sodium soy sauce
- 1 tablespoon hoisin sauce
- 1 tablespoon rice vinegar
- 1/2 cup water chestnuts, chopped
- 1/4 cup green onions, sliced
- 1 head butter lettuce, leaves separated

Instructions:
1. In a large skillet, heat the olive oil over medium heat. Add the garlic and ginger, and sauté for 1-2 minutes until fragrant.
2. Add the ground chicken and cook until browned, about 5-7 minutes.
3. Stir in the soy sauce, hoisin sauce, and rice vinegar. Cook for another 2-3 minutes.
4. Add the chopped water chestnuts and green onions, and cook for 1-2 minutes.
5. Remove from heat and let cool slightly.
6. Spoon the chicken mixture into the lettuce leaves.
7. Serve immediately.

Nutrition Info (per serving):
- Calories: 200
- Protein: 24g
- Carbohydrates: 8g
- Fat: 8g
- Fiber: 2g
- Sugar: 3g

Serves: 4
Cooking Time: 20 minutes

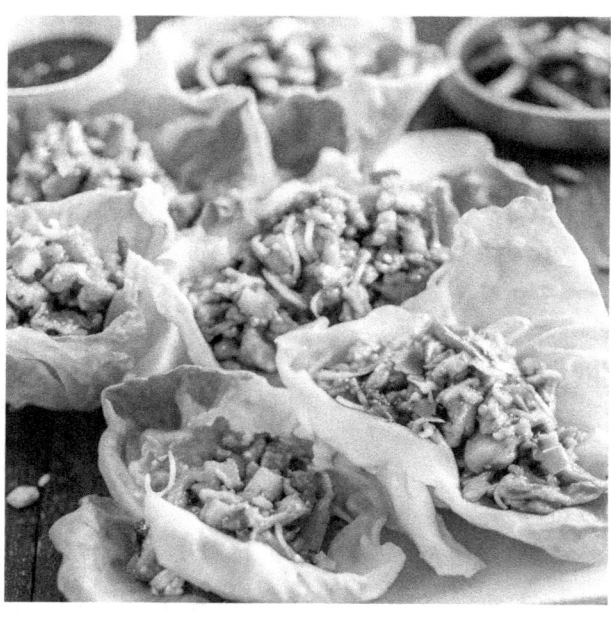

21. Chicken Veggie Stir Fry

Ingredients:
- 1 pound boneless, skinless chicken breast, cut into thin strips
- 1 tablespoon olive oil
- 2 cloves garlic, minced
- 1 tablespoon fresh ginger, grated
- 1 red bell pepper, sliced
- 1 yellow bell pepper, sliced
- 1 cup broccoli florets
- 1 cup snap peas
- 1/4 cup low-sodium soy sauce
- 1 tablespoon rice vinegar
- 1 tablespoon honey
- 1/2 teaspoon ground black pepper

Instructions:
1. In a small bowl, whisk together the soy sauce, rice vinegar, honey, and ground black pepper. Set aside.
2. Heat the olive oil in a large skillet or wok over medium-high heat.
3. Add the chicken strips and cook for 4-5 minutes until browned and cooked through. Remove from the skillet and set aside.
4. In the same skillet, add the garlic and ginger, and sauté for 1-2 minutes until fragrant.
5. Add the bell peppers, broccoli, and snap peas, and stir-fry for 3-4 minutes until tender-crisp.
6. Return the chicken to the skillet and pour the soy sauce mixture over the top. Stir to coat and cook for another 2 minutes.
7. Serve immediately.

Nutrition Info (per serving):
- Calories: 260
- Protein: 28g
- Carbohydrates: 15g
- Fat: 9g
- Fiber: 4g
- Sugar: 9g

Serves: 4
Cooking Time: 20 minutes

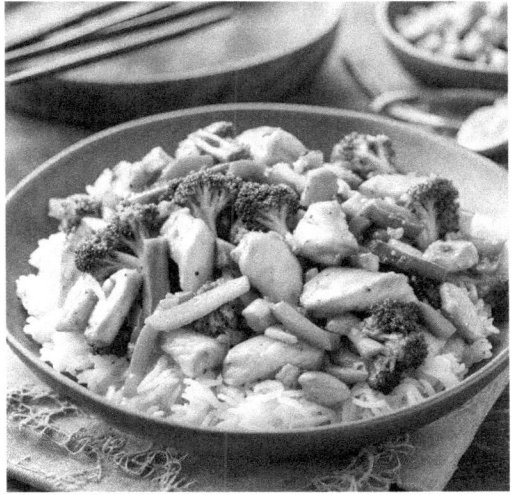

22. Baked Chicken with Rosemary and Thyme

Ingredients:
- 4 boneless, skinless chicken breasts (about 6 ounces each)
- 2 tablespoons olive oil
- 2 cloves garlic, minced
- 1 tablespoon fresh rosemary, chopped
- 1 tablespoon fresh thyme, chopped
- 1 lemon, thinly sliced
- 1/2 teaspoon ground black pepper

Instructions:
1. Preheat the oven to 375°F (190°C).
2. In a small bowl, mix together the olive oil, garlic, rosemary, thyme, and ground black pepper.
3. Rub the mixture all over the chicken breasts.
4. Place the chicken breasts in a baking dish and top with lemon slices.
5. Bake for 25-30 minutes, or until the chicken is cooked through and the internal temperature reaches 165°F (74°C).
6. Remove from the oven and let rest for 5 minutes before serving.
7. Serve immediately.

Nutrition Info (per serving):
- Calories: 250
- Protein: 36g
- Carbohydrates: 3g
- Fat: 10g
- Fiber: 1g
- Sugar: 1g

Serves: 4
Cooking Time: 30 minutes

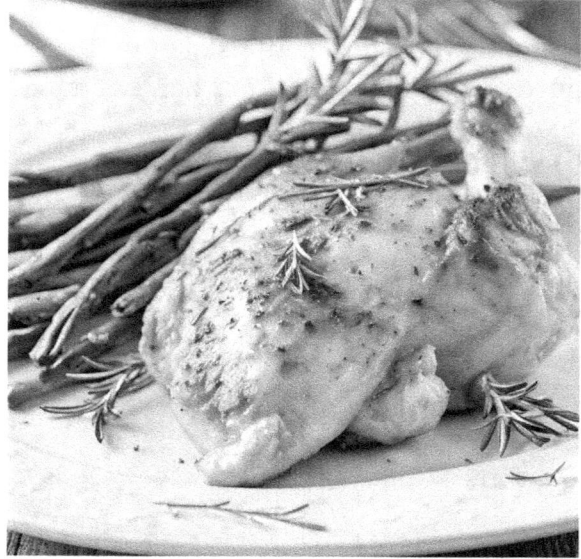

23. Grilled Chicken Caesar Salad

Ingredients:
- 4 boneless, skinless chicken breasts (about 6 ounces each)
- 2 tablespoons olive oil
- 1 teaspoon garlic powder
- 1/2 teaspoon ground black pepper
- 1 head Romaine lettuce, chopped
- 1/4 cup grated Parmesan cheese
- 1 cup cherry tomatoes, halved
- 1/4 cup Caesar dressing (low-fat or homemade)

Instructions:
1. Preheat the grill to medium-high heat.
2. In a small bowl, mix together the olive oil, garlic powder, and ground black pepper.
3. Brush the chicken breasts with the olive oil mixture.
4. Grill the chicken breasts for 5-7 minutes on each side, or until the internal temperature reaches 165°F (74°C).
5. Remove from the grill and let rest for 5 minutes before slicing.
6. In a large bowl, combine the Romaine lettuce, Parmesan cheese, and cherry tomatoes.
7. Top with the grilled chicken slices and drizzle with Caesar dressing.
8. Toss gently to combine.
9. Serve immediately.

Nutrition Info (per serving):
- Calories: 320
- Protein: 38g
- Carbohydrates: 8g
- Fat: 16g
- Fiber: 2g
- Sugar: 3g

Serves: 4
Cooking Time: 20 minutes

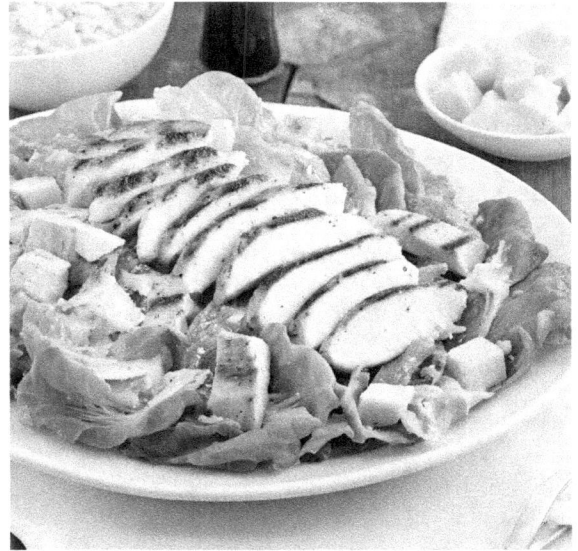

24. Chicken and Sweet Corn Soup

Ingredients:
- 1 pound boneless, skinless chicken breast, diced
- 1 tablespoon olive oil
- 1 onion, finely chopped
- 2 cloves garlic, minced
- 4 cups low-sodium chicken broth
- 1 cup fresh or frozen sweet corn kernels
- 1 carrot, diced
- 1 celery stalk, diced
- 1/2 teaspoon ground black pepper
- 1/4 cup fresh parsley, chopped

Instructions:
1. In a large pot, heat the olive oil over medium heat. Add the onion and garlic, and sauté for 3-4 minutes until softened.
2. Add the diced chicken and cook until browned, about 5-7 minutes.
3. Stir in the chicken broth, sweet corn, carrot, celery, and ground black pepper. Bring to a boil.
4. Reduce heat and simmer for 20 minutes, or until the vegetables are tender.
5. Remove from heat and stir in the fresh parsley.
6. Serve immediately.

Nutrition Info (per serving):
- Calories: 220
- Protein: 26g
- Carbohydrates: 16g
- Fat: 7g
- Fiber: 3g
- Sugar: 6g

Serves: 4
Cooking Time: 30 minutes

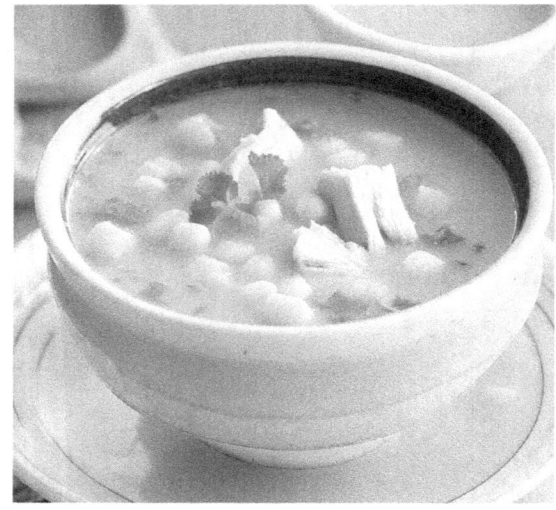

25. Roasted Chicken with Apples and Onions

Ingredients:
- 4 boneless, skinless chicken breasts (about 6 ounces each)
- 2 tablespoons olive oil
- 2 apples, cored and sliced
- 1 onion, sliced
- 1 tablespoon fresh thyme, chopped
- 1/2 teaspoon ground black pepper
- 1/4 cup low-sodium chicken broth

Instructions:
1. Preheat the oven to 375°F (190°C).
2. In a large skillet, heat the olive oil over medium heat. Add the chicken breasts and cook until browned, about 3-4 minutes on each side.
3. Remove the chicken from the skillet and set aside.
4. In the same skillet, add the apples, onion, thyme, and ground black pepper. Sauté for 5 minutes until softened.
5. Place the chicken breasts back in the skillet and pour the chicken broth over the top.
6. Transfer the skillet to the oven and roast for 25-30 minutes, or until the chicken is cooked through and the internal temperature reaches 165°F (74°C).
7. Remove from the oven and let rest for 5 minutes before serving.
8. Serve immediately.

Nutrition Info (per serving):
- Calories: 280
- Protein: 36g
- Carbohydrates: 14g
- Fat: 10g
- Fiber: 3g
- Sugar: 10g

Serves: 4
Cooking Time: 30 minutes

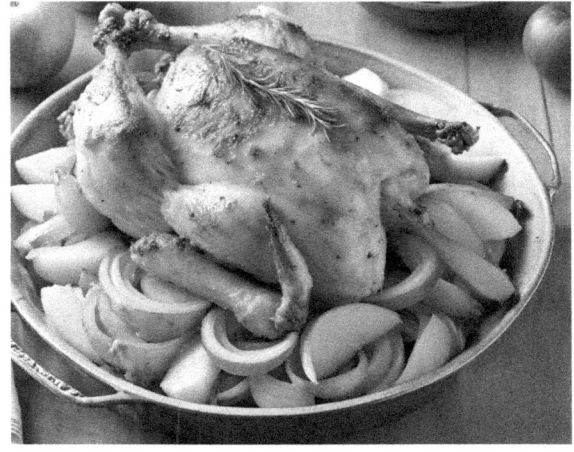

26. Steamed Chicken with Ginger and Scallions

Ingredients:
- 1 pound boneless, skinless chicken breast, cut into thin strips
- 2 tablespoons low-sodium soy sauce
- 1 tablespoon fresh ginger, grated
- 2 cloves garlic, minced
- 1 tablespoon sesame oil
- 1/4 cup green onions, sliced
- 1/2 teaspoon ground black pepper

Instructions:
1. In a bowl, combine the soy sauce, ginger, garlic, sesame oil, and ground black pepper.
2. Add the chicken strips to the bowl and toss to coat. Let marinate for 15 minutes.
3. Bring a pot of water to a boil and place a steamer basket over the pot.
4. Arrange the marinated chicken strips in the steamer basket.
5. Cover and steam for 10-12 minutes, or until the chicken is cooked through.
6. Remove from the steamer and place on a serving plate.
7. Garnish with sliced green onions.
8. Serve immediately.

Nutrition Info (per serving):
- Calories: 220
- Protein: 28g
- Carbohydrates: 3g
- Fat: 10g
- Fiber: 1g
- Sugar: 1g

Serves: 4
Cooking Time: 20 minutes

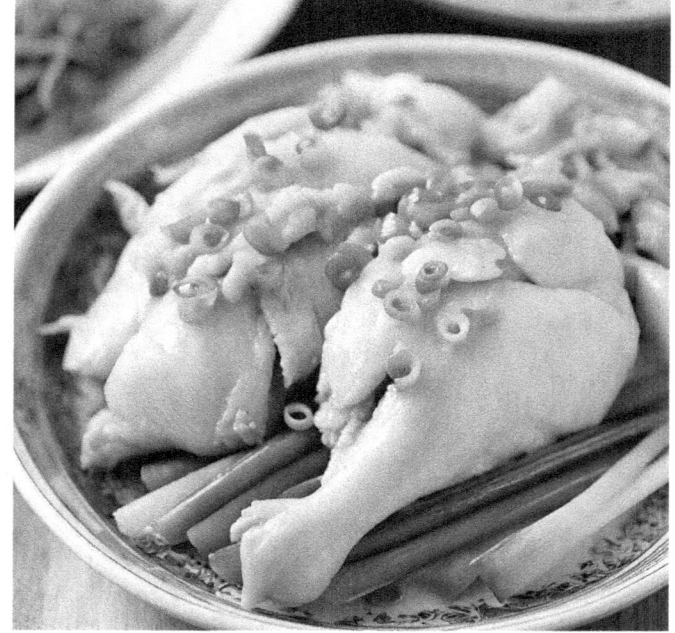

27. Grilled Chicken with Herb Marinade

Ingredients:
- 4 boneless, skinless chicken breasts (about 6 ounces each)
- 2 tablespoons olive oil
- 1 tablespoon fresh lemon juice
- 2 cloves garlic, minced
- 1 tablespoon fresh basil, chopped
- 1 tablespoon fresh parsley, chopped
- 1/2 teaspoon ground black pepper

Instructions:
1. In a small bowl, mix together the olive oil, lemon juice, garlic, basil, parsley, and ground black pepper.
2. Place the chicken breasts in a shallow dish and pour the marinade over them, turning to coat both sides. Let marinate in the refrigerator for at least 30 minutes.
3. Preheat the grill to medium-high heat.
4. Grill the chicken breasts for 5-7 minutes on each side, or until the internal temperature reaches 165°F (74°C).
5. Remove from the grill and let rest for 5 minutes before serving.
6. Serve immediately.

Nutrition Info (per serving):
- Calories: 250
- Protein: 36g
- Carbohydrates: 2g
- Fat: 10g
- Fiber: 1g
- Sugar: 1g

Serves: 4
Cooking Time: 20 minutes (plus marinating time)

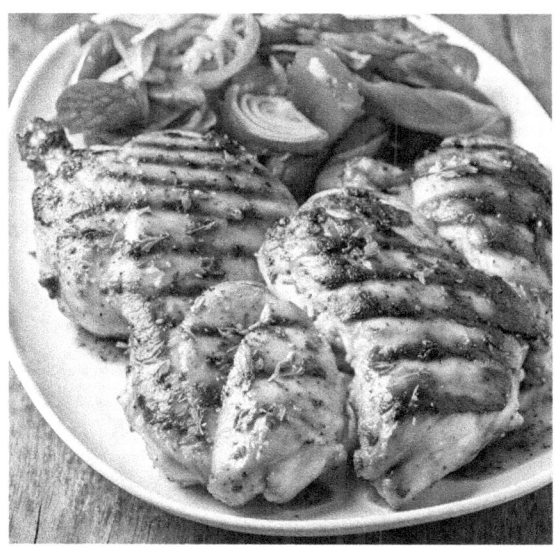

Soup and Stew Recipes

1. Lemon and Dill White Fish Stew
Ingredients:
- 1 pound white fish fillets (such as cod or haddock), cut into chunks
- 2 tablespoons olive oil
- 1 onion, chopped
- 2 cloves garlic, minced
- 4 cups low-sodium fish or vegetable broth
- 2 carrots, sliced
- 2 celery stalks, sliced
- 1 potato, peeled and diced
- 1 cup diced tomatoes (canned, no added salt)
- 1 tablespoon fresh dill, chopped
- 1 lemon, juiced and zested
- 1/2 teaspoon ground black pepper

Instructions:
1. In a large pot, heat the olive oil over medium heat. Add the onion and garlic, and sauté for 3-4 minutes until softened.
2. Add the carrots, celery, and potato, and cook for another 5 minutes, stirring occasionally.
3. Pour in the broth and diced tomatoes. Bring to a boil, then reduce heat and simmer for 20 minutes, or until the vegetables are tender.
4. Add the fish chunks, lemon juice, lemon zest, dill, and ground black pepper. Simmer for another 10 minutes, or until the fish is cooked through and flakes easily with a fork.
5. Remove from heat and serve immediately.

Nutrition Info (per serving):
- Calories: 220
- Protein: 25g
- Carbohydrates: 22g
- Fat: 6g
- Fiber: 4g
- Sugar: 6g

Serves: 4
Cooking Time: 40 minutes

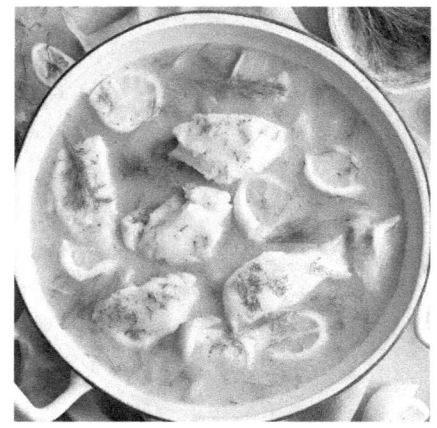

2. Garbanzo Bean and Vegetable Soup

Ingredients:
- 1 tablespoon olive oil
- 1 onion, chopped
- 2 cloves garlic, minced
- 2 carrots, sliced
- 2 celery stalks, sliced
- 1 zucchini, diced
- 1 red bell pepper, chopped
- 1 can (15 ounces) garbanzo beans, rinsed and drained
- 4 cups low-sodium vegetable broth
- 1 can (15 ounces) diced tomatoes (no added salt)
- 1 teaspoon dried thyme
- 1/2 teaspoon ground black pepper
- 1/4 cup fresh parsley, chopped

Instructions:
1. In a large pot, heat the olive oil over medium heat. Add the onion and garlic, and sauté for 3-4 minutes until softened.
2. Add the carrots, celery, zucchini, and red bell pepper. Cook for another 5 minutes, stirring occasionally.
3. Stir in the garbanzo beans, vegetable broth, diced tomatoes, dried thyme, and ground black pepper. Bring to a boil.
4. Reduce heat and simmer for 25-30 minutes, or until the vegetables are tender.
5. Remove from heat and stir in the fresh parsley.
6. Serve immediately.

Nutrition Info (per serving):
- Calories: 200
- Protein: 7g
- Carbohydrates: 33g
- Fat: 5g
- Fiber: 8g
- Sugar: 10g

Serves: 6
Cooking Time: 40 minutes

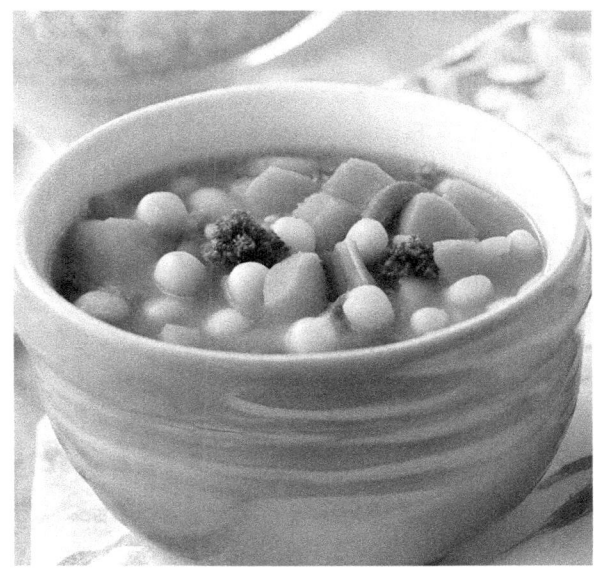

3. Jerusalem Artichoke Soup

Ingredients:
- 2 tablespoons olive oil
- 1 onion, chopped
- 2 cloves garlic, minced
- 1 pound Jerusalem artichokes, peeled and diced
- 2 potatoes, peeled and diced
- 4 cups low-sodium vegetable broth
- 1 teaspoon dried thyme
- 1/2 teaspoon ground black pepper
- 1/2 cup low-fat milk or unsweetened almond milk
- 1/4 cup fresh chives, chopped

Instructions:
1. In a large pot, heat the olive oil over medium heat. Add the onion and garlic, and sauté for 3-4 minutes until softened.
2. Add the Jerusalem artichokes and potatoes. Cook for another 5 minutes, stirring occasionally.
3. Pour in the vegetable broth, dried thyme, and ground black pepper. Bring to a boil, then reduce heat and simmer for 25-30 minutes, or until the vegetables are tender.
4. Use an immersion blender to puree the soup until smooth. Alternatively, transfer the soup to a blender in batches and blend until smooth.
5. Stir in the milk and heat gently for another 5 minutes.
6. Remove from heat and stir in the fresh chives.
7. Serve immediately.

Nutrition Info (per serving):
- Calories: 220
- Protein: 5g
- Carbohydrates: 36g
- Fat: 7g
- Fiber: 6g
- Sugar: 5g

Serves: 4
Cooking Time: 45 minutes

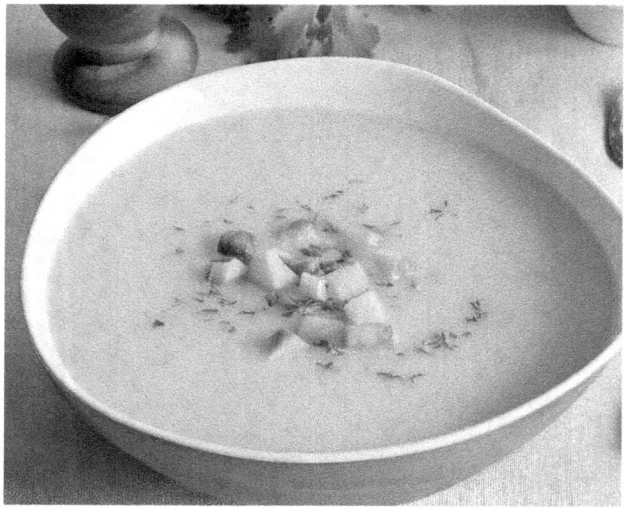

4. Artichoke and Potato Stew

Ingredients:
- 2 tablespoons olive oil
- 1 onion, chopped
- 2 cloves garlic, minced
- 4 cups low-sodium vegetable broth
- 4 potatoes, peeled and diced
- 2 cups frozen artichoke hearts, thawed and chopped
- 2 carrots, sliced
- 2 celery stalks, sliced
- 1 can (15 ounces) diced tomatoes (no added salt)
- 1 teaspoon dried basil
- 1/2 teaspoon ground black pepper
- 1/4 cup fresh parsley, chopped

Instructions:
1. In a large pot, heat the olive oil over medium heat. Add the onion and garlic, and sauté for 3-4 minutes until softened.
2. Add the potatoes, artichoke hearts, carrots, and celery. Cook for another 5 minutes, stirring occasionally.
3. Pour in the vegetable broth and diced tomatoes. Stir in the dried basil and ground black pepper. Bring to a boil.
4. Reduce heat and simmer for 30 minutes, or until the vegetables are tender.
5. Remove from heat and stir in the fresh parsley.
6. Serve immediately.

Nutrition Info (per serving):
- Calories: 230
- Protein: 5g
- Carbohydrates: 40g
- Fat: 7g
- Fiber: 8g
- Sugar: 8g

Serves: 6
Cooking Time: 40 minutes

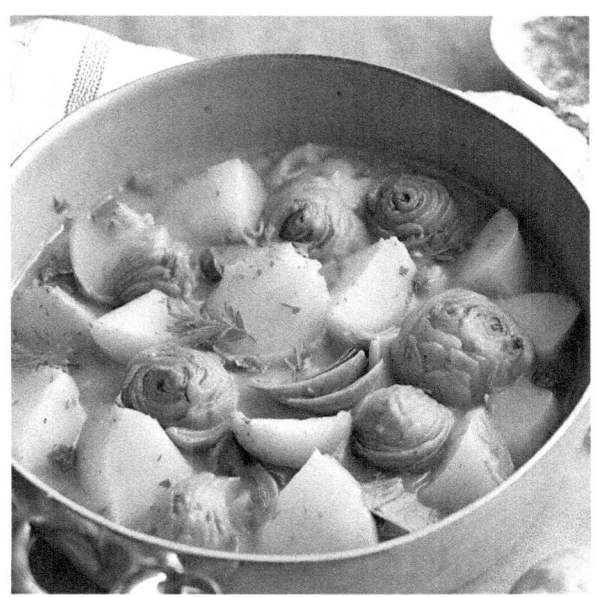

5. Corn and Zucchini Chowder

Ingredients:
- 1 tablespoon olive oil
- 1 onion, chopped
- 2 cloves garlic, minced
- 3 cups fresh or frozen corn kernels
- 2 zucchinis, diced
- 2 potatoes, peeled and diced
- 4 cups low-sodium vegetable broth
- 1 cup low-fat milk or unsweetened almond milk
- 1 teaspoon dried thyme
- 1/2 teaspoon ground black pepper
- 1/4 cup fresh parsley, chopped

Instructions:
1. In a large pot, heat the olive oil over medium heat. Add the onion and garlic, and sauté for 3-4 minutes until softened.
2. Add the corn, zucchinis, and potatoes. Cook for another 5 minutes, stirring occasionally.
3. Pour in the vegetable broth and stir in the dried thyme and ground black pepper. Bring to a boil.
4. Reduce heat and simmer for 20-25 minutes, or until the vegetables are tender.
5. Use an immersion blender to puree the soup slightly, leaving some chunks for texture.
6. Stir in the milk and heat gently for another 5 minutes.
7. Remove from heat and stir in the fresh parsley.
8. Serve immediately.

Nutrition Info (per serving):
- Calories: 220
- Protein: 6g
- Carbohydrates: 38g
- Fat: 6g
- Fiber: 6g
- Sugar: 8g

Serves: 6
Cooking Time: 35 minutes

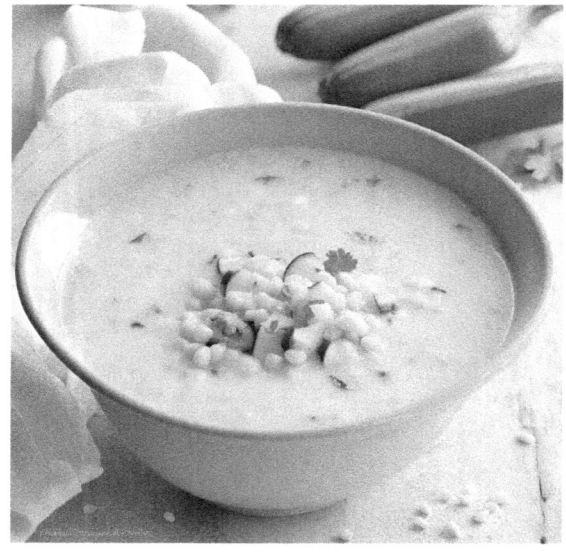

6. Black Bean Soup with Cilantro

Ingredients:
- 1 tablespoon olive oil
- 1 onion, chopped
- 2 cloves garlic, minced
- 2 carrots, diced
- 2 celery stalks, diced
- 2 cans (15 ounces each) black beans, rinsed and drained
- 4 cups low-sodium vegetable broth
- 1 teaspoon ground cumin
- 1/2 teaspoon ground black pepper
- 1/4 cup fresh cilantro, chopped
- 1 tablespoon fresh lime juice

Instructions:
1. In a large pot, heat the olive oil over medium heat. Add the onion and garlic, and sauté for 3-4 minutes until softened.
2. Add the carrots and celery, and cook for another 5 minutes, stirring occasionally.
3. Stir in the black beans, vegetable broth, ground cumin, and ground black pepper. Bring to a boil.
4. Reduce heat and simmer for 20 minutes.
5. Use an immersion blender to puree the soup slightly, leaving some beans whole for texture.
6. Stir in the fresh cilantro and lime juice.
7. Remove from heat and serve immediately.

Nutrition Info (per serving):
- Calories: 200
- Protein: 10g
- Carbohydrates: 36g
- Fat: 5g
- Fiber: 10g
- Sugar: 4g

Serves: 6
Cooking Time: 30 minutes

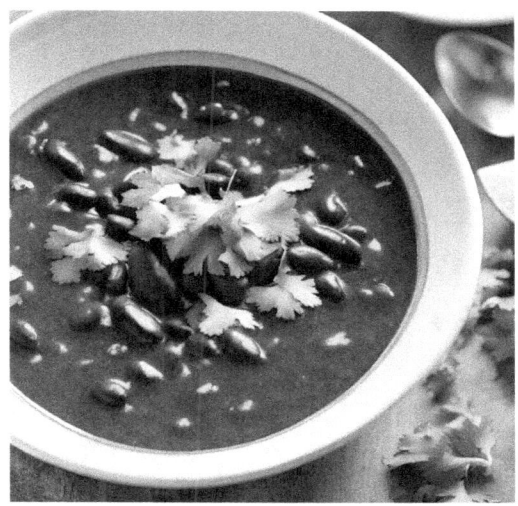

7. Watercress and Pea Soup

Ingredients:
- 1 tablespoon olive oil
- 1 onion, chopped
- 2 cloves garlic, minced
- 4 cups low-sodium vegetable broth
- 2 cups fresh or frozen peas
- 2 cups fresh watercress, chopped
- 1 potato, peeled and diced
- 1 teaspoon dried thyme
- 1/2 teaspoon ground black pepper
- 1/4 cup fresh mint, chopped

Instructions:
1. In a large pot, heat the olive oil over medium heat. Add the onion and garlic, and sauté for 3-4 minutes until softened.
2. Add the vegetable broth, peas, watercress, and potato. Stir in the dried thyme and ground black pepper. Bring to a boil.
3. Reduce heat and simmer for 20-25 minutes, or until the vegetables are tender.
4. Use an immersion blender to puree the soup until smooth.
5. Remove from heat and stir in the fresh mint.
6. Serve immediately.

Nutrition Info (per serving):
- Calories: 180
- Protein: 6g
- Carbohydrates: 30g
- Fat: 5g
- Fiber: 6g
- Sugar: 7g

Serves: 6
Cooking Time: 30 minutes

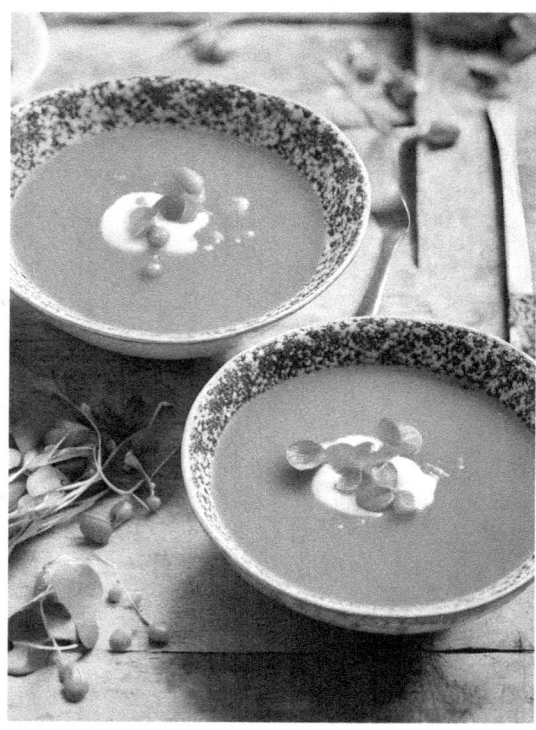

8. Beet and Cabbage Borscht

Ingredients:
- 1 tablespoon olive oil
- 1 onion, chopped
- 2 cloves garlic, minced
- 3 beets, peeled and grated
- 2 carrots, grated
- 1 potato, peeled and diced
- 4 cups low-sodium vegetable broth
- 2 cups shredded cabbage
- 1 teaspoon dried dill
- 1/2 teaspoon ground black pepper
- 2 tablespoons fresh lemon juice
- 1/4 cup fresh dill, chopped

Instructions:
1. In a large pot, heat the olive oil over medium heat. Add the onion and garlic, and sauté for 3-4 minutes until softened.
2. Add the beets, carrots, and potato. Cook for another 5 minutes, stirring occasionally.
3. Pour in the vegetable broth and stir in the shredded cabbage, dried dill, and ground black pepper. Bring to a boil.
4. Reduce heat and simmer for 25-30 minutes, or until the vegetables are tender.
5. Remove from heat and stir in the lemon juice and fresh dill.
6. Serve immediately.

Nutrition Info (per serving):
- Calories: 190
- Protein: 4g
- Carbohydrates: 35g
- Fat: 5g
- Fiber: 8g
- Sugar: 14g

Serves: 6
Cooking Time: 35 minutes

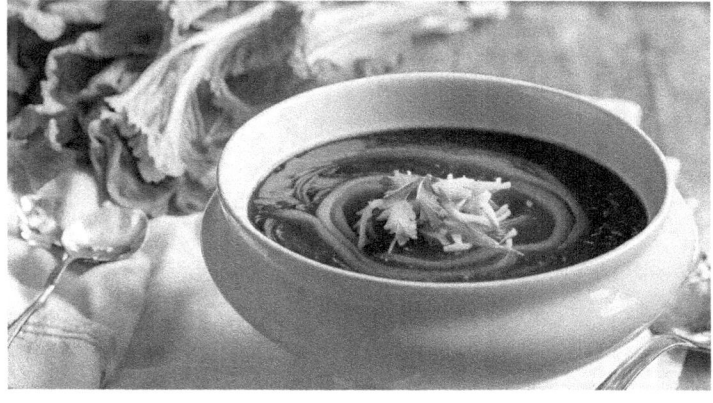

9. Green Bean and Potato Soup

Ingredients:
- 1 tablespoon olive oil
- 1 onion, chopped
- 2 cloves garlic, minced
- 3 potatoes, peeled and diced
- 4 cups low-sodium vegetable broth
- 2 cups green beans, trimmed and cut into 1-inch pieces
- 1 teaspoon dried thyme
- 1/2 teaspoon ground black pepper
- 1/4 cup fresh parsley, chopped

Instructions:
1. In a large pot, heat the olive oil over medium heat. Add the onion and garlic, and sauté for 3-4 minutes until softened.
2. Add the potatoes and cook for another 5 minutes, stirring occasionally.
3. Pour in the vegetable broth and bring to a boil. Reduce heat and simmer for 15 minutes.
4. Add the green beans, dried thyme, and ground black pepper. Simmer for another 10-15 minutes, or until the vegetables are tender.
5. Remove from heat and stir in the fresh parsley.
6. Serve immediately.

Nutrition Info (per serving):
- Calories: 180
- Protein: 4g
- Carbohydrates: 33g
- Fat: 5g
- Fiber: 6g
- Sugar: 5g

Serves: 6
Cooking Time: 30 minutes

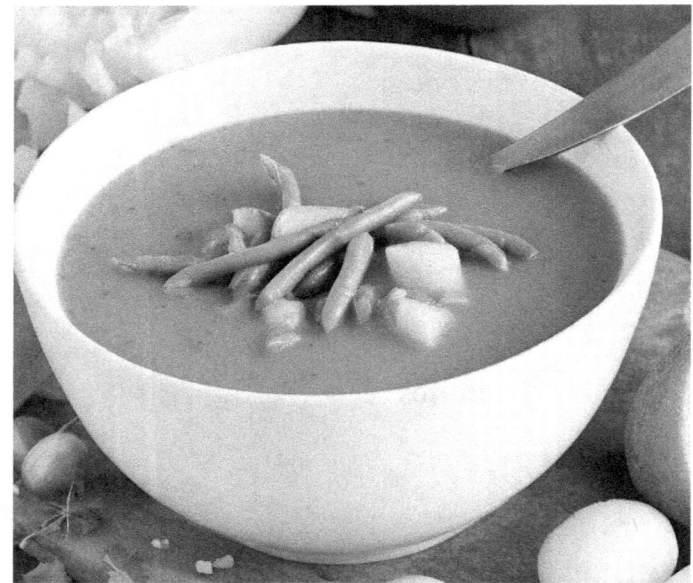

10. Cauliflower and Chickpea Soup

Ingredients:
- 1 tablespoon olive oil
- 1 onion, chopped
- 2 cloves garlic, minced
- 1 head cauliflower, chopped
- 1 can (15 ounces) chickpeas, rinsed and drained
- 4 cups low-sodium vegetable broth
- 1 teaspoon ground cumin
- 1/2 teaspoon ground black pepper
- 1/4 cup fresh parsley, chopped

Instructions:
1. In a large pot, heat the olive oil over medium heat. Add the onion and garlic, and sauté for 3-4 minutes until softened.
2. Add the cauliflower and cook for another 5 minutes, stirring occasionally.
3. Stir in the chickpeas, vegetable broth, ground cumin, and ground black pepper. Bring to a boil.
4. Reduce heat and simmer for 20-25 minutes, or until the cauliflower is tender.
5. Use an immersion blender to puree the soup until smooth, leaving some chunks if desired.
6. Remove from heat and stir in the fresh parsley.
7. Serve immediately.

Nutrition Info (per serving):
- Calories: 180
- Protein: 7g
- Carbohydrates: 28g
- Fat: 6g
- Fiber: 8g
- Sugar: 5g

Serves: 4
Cooking Time: 30 minutes

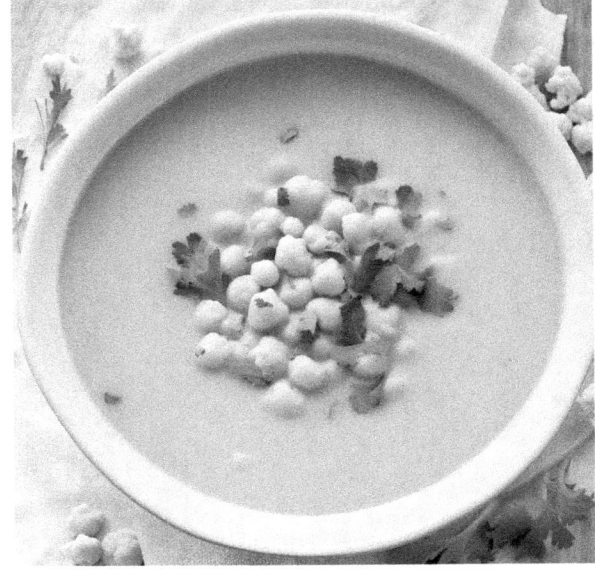

11. Turnip and Parsnip Soup

Ingredients:
- 1 tablespoon olive oil
- 1 onion, chopped
- 2 cloves garlic, minced
- 2 turnips, peeled and diced
- 2 parsnips, peeled and diced
- 4 cups low-sodium vegetable broth
- 1 teaspoon dried thyme
- 1/2 teaspoon ground black pepper
- 1/4 cup fresh chives, chopped

Instructions:
1. In a large pot, heat the olive oil over medium heat. Add the onion and garlic, and sauté for 3-4 minutes until softened.
2. Add the turnips and parsnips. Cook for another 5 minutes, stirring occasionally.
3. Pour in the vegetable broth and stir in the dried thyme and ground black pepper. Bring to a boil.
4. Reduce heat and simmer for 25-30 minutes, or until the vegetables are tender.
5. Use an immersion blender to puree the soup until smooth.
6. Remove from heat and stir in the fresh chives.
7. Serve immediately.

Nutrition Info (per serving):
- Calories: 170
- Protein: 3g
- Carbohydrates: 29g
- Fat: 5g
- Fiber: 6g
- Sugar: 10g

Serves: 4
Cooking Time: 35 minutes

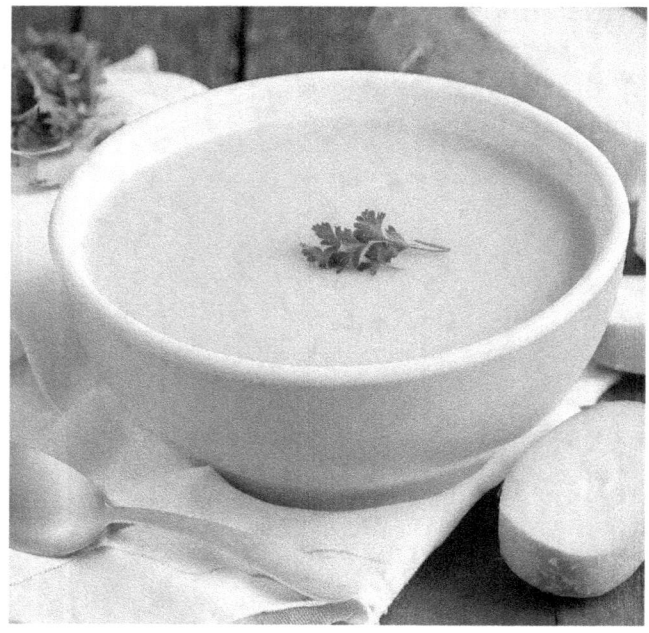

12. Mushroom and Barley Soup

Ingredients:
- 1 tablespoon olive oil
- 1 onion, chopped
- 2 cloves garlic, minced
- 2 cups mushrooms, sliced
- 1 cup pearl barley, rinsed
- 4 cups low-sodium vegetable broth
- 1 teaspoon dried thyme
- 1/2 teaspoon ground black pepper
- 1/4 cup fresh parsley, chopped

Instructions:
1. In a large pot, heat the olive oil over medium heat. Add the onion and garlic, and sauté for 3-4 minutes until softened.
2. Add the mushrooms and cook for another 5 minutes, stirring occasionally.
3. Stir in the barley, vegetable broth, dried thyme, and ground black pepper. Bring to a boil.
4. Reduce heat and simmer for 40-45 minutes, or until the barley is tender.
5. Remove from heat and stir in the fresh parsley.
6. Serve immediately.

Nutrition Info (per serving):
- Calories: 200
- Protein: 6g
- Carbohydrates: 40g
- Fat: 5g
- Fiber: 7g
- Sugar: 6g

Serves: 4
Cooking Time: 50 minutes

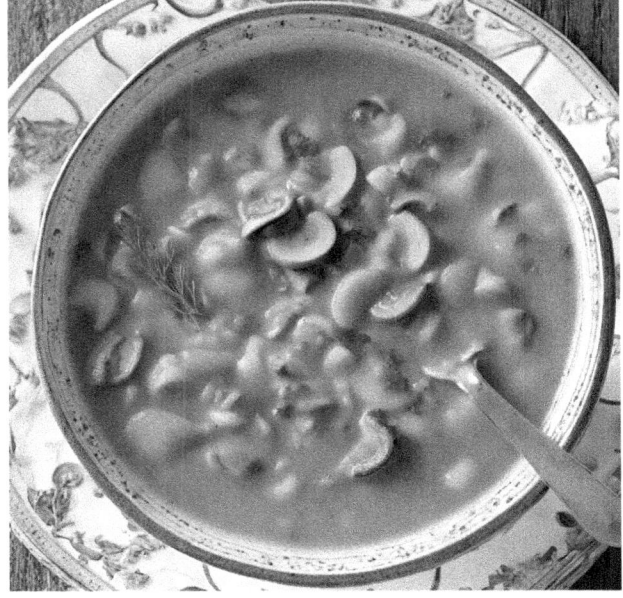

13. Fennel and Bean Stew

Ingredients:
- 1 tablespoon olive oil
- 1 onion, chopped
- 2 cloves garlic, minced
- 2 fennel bulbs, trimmed and sliced
- 2 carrots, sliced
- 1 can (15 ounces) cannellini beans, rinsed and drained
- 4 cups low-sodium vegetable broth
- 1 teaspoon dried oregano
- 1/2 teaspoon ground black pepper
- 1/4 cup fresh basil, chopped

Instructions:
1. In a large pot, heat the olive oil over medium heat. Add the onion and garlic, and sauté for 3-4 minutes until softened.
2. Add the fennel and carrots. Cook for another 5 minutes, stirring occasionally.
3. Stir in the beans, vegetable broth, dried oregano, and ground black pepper. Bring to a boil.
4. Reduce heat and simmer for 30 minutes, or until the vegetables are tender.
5. Remove from heat and stir in the fresh basil.
6. Serve immediately.

Nutrition Info (per serving):
- Calories: 220
- Protein: 7g
- Carbohydrates: 35g
- Fat: 6g
- Fiber: 9g
- Sugar: 7g

Serves: 4
Cooking Time: 40 minutes

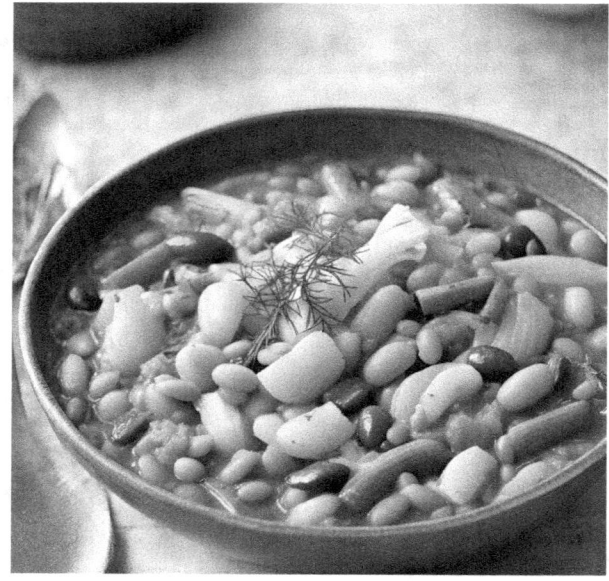

14. Eggplant and Tomato Stew

Ingredients:
- 1 tablespoon olive oil
- 1 onion, chopped
- 2 cloves garlic, minced
- 1 large eggplant, diced
- 2 cups diced tomatoes (canned, no added salt)
- 2 zucchini, sliced
- 1 red bell pepper, chopped
- 4 cups low-sodium vegetable broth
- 1 teaspoon dried basil
- 1/2 teaspoon ground black pepper
- 1/4 cup fresh parsley, chopped

Instructions:
1. In a large pot, heat the olive oil over medium heat. Add the onion and garlic, and sauté for 3-4 minutes until softened.
2. Add the eggplant and cook for another 5 minutes, stirring occasionally.
3. Stir in the tomatoes, zucchini, red bell pepper, vegetable broth, dried basil, and ground black pepper. Bring to a boil.
4. Reduce heat and simmer for 30 minutes, or until the vegetables are tender.
5. Remove from heat and stir in the fresh parsley.
6. Serve immediately.

Nutrition Info (per serving):
- Calories: 180
- Protein: 5g
- Carbohydrates: 32g
- Fat: 5g
- Fiber: 8g
- Sugar: 14g

Serves: 4
Cooking Time: 40 minutes

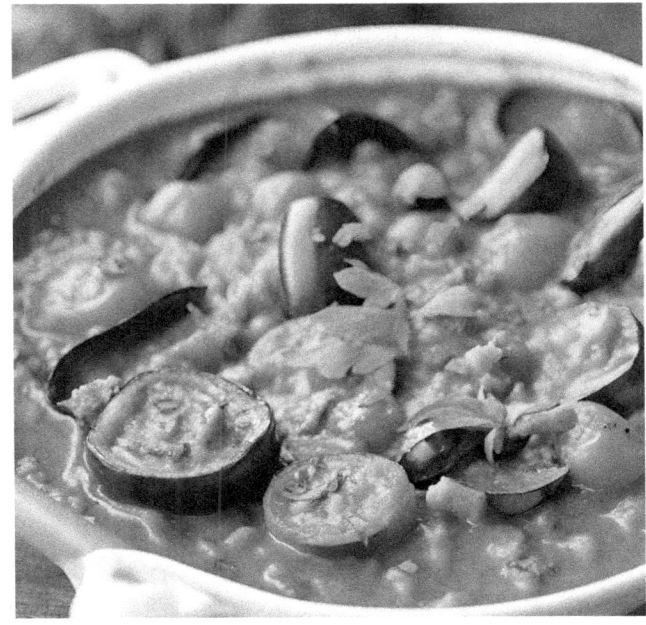

15. Broccoli and Lentil Soup

Ingredients:
- 1 tablespoon olive oil
- 1 onion, chopped
- 2 cloves garlic, minced
- 1 head of broccoli, chopped
- 1 cup lentils, rinsed
- 4 cups low-sodium vegetable broth
- 2 carrots, sliced
- 2 celery stalks, sliced
- 1 teaspoon dried thyme
- 1/2 teaspoon ground black pepper
- 1/4 cup fresh parsley, chopped

Instructions:
1. In a large pot, heat the olive oil over medium heat. Add the onion and garlic, and sauté for 3-4 minutes until softened.
2. Add the carrots, celery, broccoli, and lentils. Cook for another 5 minutes, stirring occasionally.
3. Pour in the vegetable broth and stir in the dried thyme and ground black pepper. Bring to a boil.
4. Reduce heat and simmer for 25-30 minutes, or until the lentils and vegetables are tender.
5. Use an immersion blender to puree the soup slightly, leaving some chunks for texture.
6. Remove from heat and stir in the fresh parsley.
7. Serve immediately.

Nutrition Info (per serving):
- Calories: 210
- Protein: 12g
- Carbohydrates: 34g
- Fat: 6g
- Fiber: 12g
- Sugar: 6g

Serves: 4
Cooking Time: 35 minutes

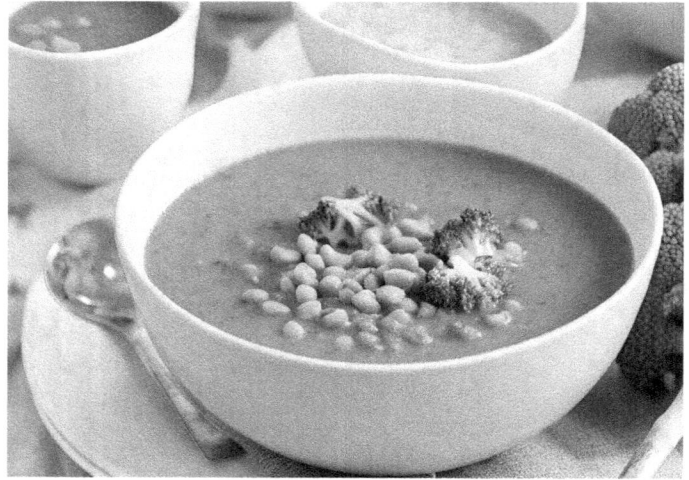

16. Chickpea and Spinach Soup

Ingredients:
- 1 tablespoon olive oil
- 1 onion, chopped
- 2 cloves garlic, minced
- 2 carrots, sliced
- 1 can (15 ounces) chickpeas, rinsed and drained
- 4 cups low-sodium vegetable broth
- 1 can (15 ounces) diced tomatoes (no added salt)
- 1 teaspoon ground cumin
- 1/2 teaspoon ground black pepper
- 4 cups fresh spinach, chopped
- 1/4 cup fresh cilantro, chopped

Instructions:
1. In a large pot, heat the olive oil over medium heat. Add the onion and garlic, and sauté for 3-4 minutes until softened.
2. Add the carrots and cook for another 5 minutes, stirring occasionally.
3. Stir in the chickpeas, vegetable broth, diced tomatoes, ground cumin, and ground black pepper. Bring to a boil.
4. Reduce heat and simmer for 20 minutes.
5. Stir in the fresh spinach and cook for another 5 minutes, until wilted.
6. Remove from heat and stir in the fresh cilantro.
7. Serve immediately.

Nutrition Info (per serving):
- Calories: 200
- Protein: 9g
- Carbohydrates: 30g
- Fat: 5g
- Fiber: 8g
- Sugar: 6g

Serves: 4
Cooking Time: 30 minutes

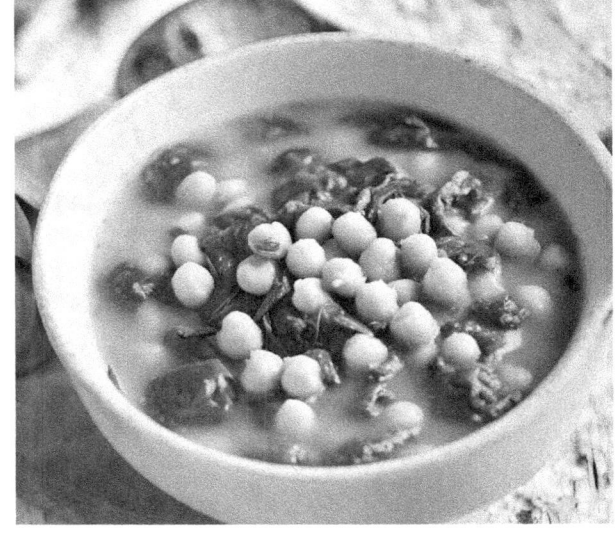

17. Asparagus and White Bean Soup

Ingredients:
- 1 tablespoon olive oil
- 1 onion, chopped
- 2 cloves garlic, minced
- 1 pound asparagus, trimmed and cut into 1-inch pieces
- 1 can (15 ounces) white beans, rinsed and drained
- 4 cups low-sodium vegetable broth
- 1 potato, peeled and diced
- 1 teaspoon dried tarragon
- 1/2 teaspoon ground black pepper
- 1/4 cup fresh dill, chopped

Instructions:
1. In a large pot, heat the olive oil over medium heat. Add the onion and garlic, and sauté for 3-4 minutes until softened.
2. Add the asparagus and potato. Cook for another 5 minutes, stirring occasionally.
3. Stir in the white beans, vegetable broth, and dried tarragon. Bring to a boil.
4. Reduce heat and simmer for 25-30 minutes, or until the vegetables are tender.
5. Use an immersion blender to puree the soup until smooth.
6. Remove from heat and stir in the fresh dill.
7. Serve immediately.

Nutrition Info (per serving):
- Calories: 190
- Protein: 8g
- Carbohydrates: 30g
- Fat: 5g
- Fiber: 8g
- Sugar: 4g

Serves: 4
Cooking Time: 35 minutes

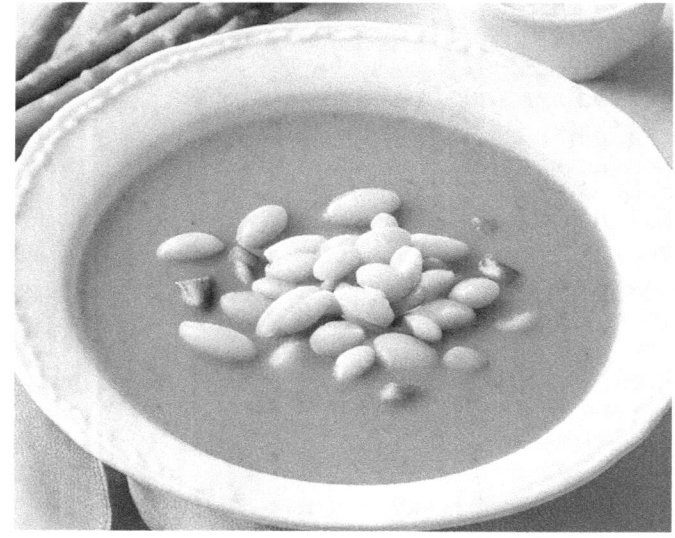

18. Quinoa and Vegetable Soup

Ingredients:
- 1 tablespoon olive oil
- 1 onion, chopped
- 2 cloves garlic, minced
- 2 carrots, sliced
- 2 celery stalks, sliced
- 1 zucchini, diced
- 1/2 cup quinoa, rinsed
- 4 cups low-sodium vegetable broth
- 1 can (15 ounces) diced tomatoes (no added salt)
- 1 teaspoon dried basil
- 1/2 teaspoon ground black pepper
- 1/4 cup fresh basil, chopped

Instructions:
1. In a large pot, heat the olive oil over medium heat. Add the onion and garlic, and sauté for 3-4 minutes until softened.
2. Add the carrots, celery, zucchini, and quinoa. Cook for another 5 minutes, stirring occasionally.
3. Stir in the vegetable broth, diced tomatoes, dried basil, and ground black pepper. Bring to a boil.
4. Reduce heat and simmer for 25-30 minutes, or until the quinoa and vegetables are tender.
5. Remove from heat and stir in the fresh basil.
6. Serve immediately.

Nutrition Info (per serving):
- Calories: 200
- Protein: 7g
- Carbohydrates: 36g
- Fat: 5g
- Fiber: 8g
- Sugar: 7g

Serves: 4
Cooking Time: 35 minutes

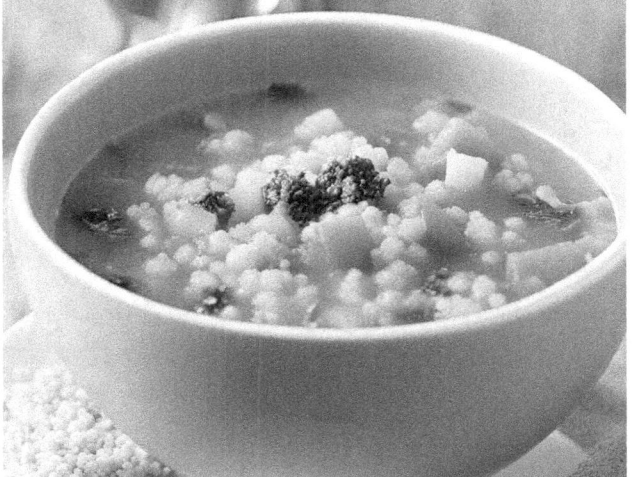

19. Bean and Swiss Chard Stew

Ingredients:
- 1 tablespoon olive oil
- 1 onion, chopped
- 2 cloves garlic, minced
- 1 bunch Swiss chard, stems removed and leaves chopped
- 2 carrots, sliced
- 1 can (15 ounces) cannellini beans, rinsed and drained
- 4 cups low-sodium vegetable broth
- 1 can (15 ounces) diced tomatoes (no added salt)
- 1 teaspoon dried oregano
- 1/2 teaspoon ground black pepper
- 1/4 cup fresh parsley, chopped

Instructions:
1. In a large pot, heat the olive oil over medium heat. Add the onion and garlic, and sauté for 3-4 minutes until softened.
2. Add the Swiss chard and carrots. Cook for another 5 minutes, stirring occasionally.
3. Stir in the beans, vegetable broth, diced tomatoes, dried oregano, and ground black pepper. Bring to a boil.
4. Reduce heat and simmer for 25-30 minutes, or until the vegetables are tender.
5. Remove from heat and stir in the fresh parsley.
6. Serve immediately.

Nutrition Info (per serving):
- Calories: 210
- Protein: 8g
- Carbohydrates: 35g
- Fat: 5g
- Fiber: 9g
- Sugar: 8g

Serves: 4
Cooking Time: 35 minutes

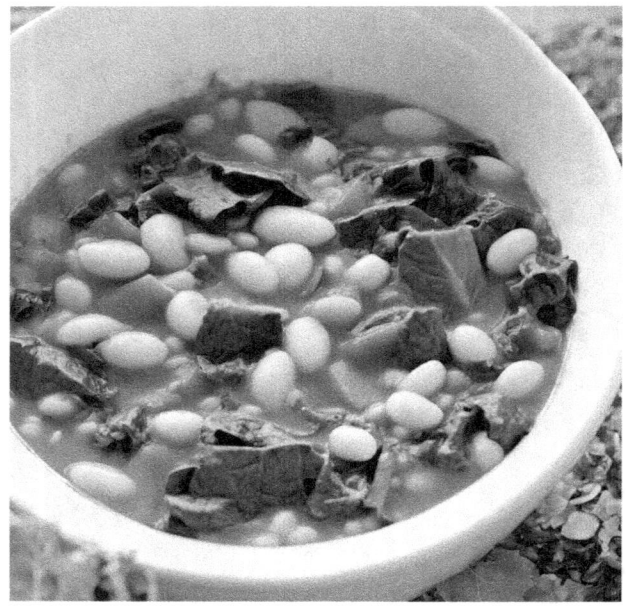

20. Red Lentil and Carrot Stew

Ingredients:
- 1 tablespoon olive oil
- 1 onion, chopped
- 2 cloves garlic, minced
- 2 cups carrots, sliced
- 1 cup red lentils, rinsed
- 4 cups low-sodium vegetable broth
- 1 teaspoon ground cumin
- 1/2 teaspoon ground coriander
- 1/2 teaspoon ground black pepper
- 1/4 cup fresh cilantro, chopped

Instructions:
1. In a large pot, heat the olive oil over medium heat. Add the onion and garlic, and sauté for 3-4 minutes until softened.
2. Add the carrots and cook for another 5 minutes, stirring occasionally.
3. Stir in the red lentils, vegetable broth, ground cumin, ground coriander, and ground black pepper. Bring to a boil.
4. Reduce heat and simmer for 25-30 minutes, or until the lentils and carrots are tender.
5. Use an immersion blender to puree the stew slightly, leaving some chunks for texture.
6. Remove from heat and stir in the fresh cilantro.
7. Serve immediately.

Nutrition Info (per serving):
- Calories: 220
- Protein: 10g
- Carbohydrates: 35g
- Fat: 5g
- Fiber: 10g
- Sugar: 7g

Serves: 4
Cooking Time: 35 minutes

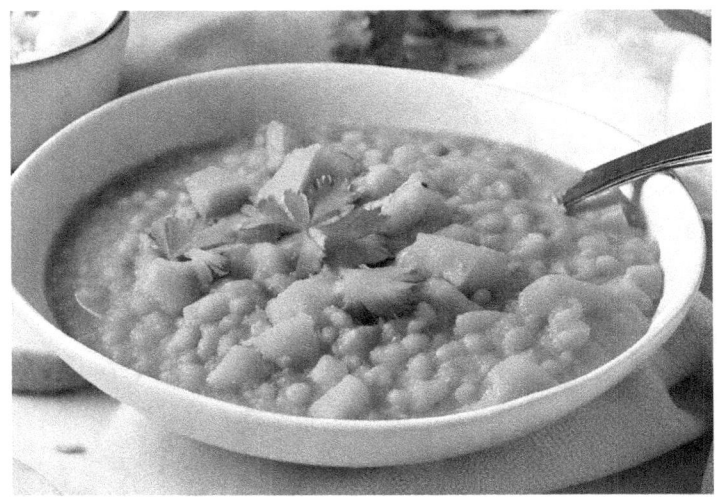

21. Sweet Potato and Lentil Soup

Ingredients:
- 1 tablespoon olive oil
- 1 onion, chopped
- 2 cloves garlic, minced
- 2 cups sweet potatoes, peeled and diced
- 1 cup red lentils, rinsed
- 4 cups low-sodium vegetable broth
- 1 teaspoon ground ginger
- 1/2 teaspoon ground cinnamon
- 1/2 teaspoon ground black pepper
- 1/4 cup fresh parsley, chopped

Instructions:
1. In a large pot, heat the olive oil over medium heat. Add the onion and garlic, and sauté for 3-4 minutes until softened.
2. Add the sweet potatoes and cook for another 5 minutes, stirring occasionally.
3. Stir in the red lentils, vegetable broth, ground ginger, ground cinnamon, and ground black pepper. Bring to a boil.
4. Reduce heat and simmer for 25-30 minutes, or until the lentils and sweet potatoes are tender.
5. Use an immersion blender to puree the soup until smooth.
6. Remove from heat and stir in the fresh parsley.
7. Serve immediately.

Nutrition Info (per serving):
- Calories: 240
- Protein: 10g
- Carbohydrates: 42g
- Fat: 5g
- Fiber: 9g
- Sugar: 8g

Serves: 4
Cooking Time: 35 minutes

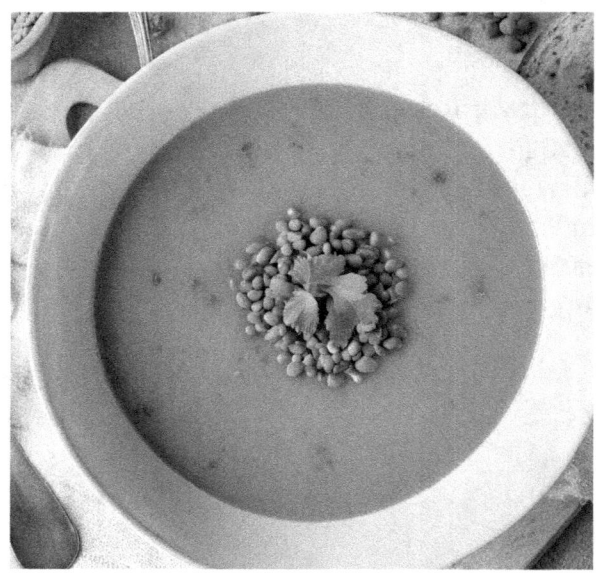

22. Kale and White Bean Soup

Ingredients:
- 1 tablespoon olive oil
- 1 onion, chopped
- 2 cloves garlic, minced
- 2 cups kale, chopped
- 1 can (15 ounces) white beans, rinsed and drained
- 4 cups low-sodium vegetable broth
- 1 potato, peeled and diced
- 1 teaspoon dried thyme
- 1/2 teaspoon ground black pepper
- 1/4 cup fresh dill, chopped

Instructions:
1. In a large pot, heat the olive oil over medium heat. Add the onion and garlic, and sauté for 3-4 minutes until softened.
2. Add the kale and cook for another 5 minutes, stirring occasionally.
3. Stir in the white beans, vegetable broth, potato, dried thyme, and ground black pepper. Bring to a boil.
4. Reduce heat and simmer for 25-30 minutes, or until the potato is tender.
5. Use an immersion blender to puree the soup slightly, leaving some chunks for texture.
6. Remove from heat and stir in the fresh dill.
7. Serve immediately.

Nutrition Info (per serving):
- Calories: 210
- Protein: 8g
- Carbohydrates: 36g
- Fat: 5g
- Fiber: 10g
- Sugar: 4g

Serves: 4
Cooking Time: 35 minutes

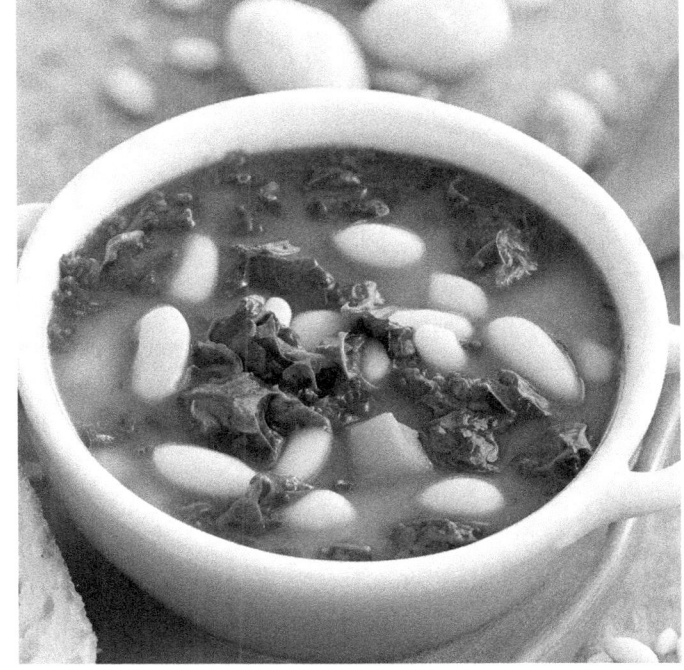

23. Pumpkin and Bean Soup

Ingredients:
- 1 tablespoon olive oil
- 1 onion, chopped
- 2 cloves garlic, minced
- 2 cups pumpkin puree (canned, no added sugar)
- 1 can (15 ounces) cannellini beans, rinsed and drained
- 4 cups low-sodium vegetable broth
- 1 teaspoon ground cumin
- 1/2 teaspoon ground black pepper
- 1/4 cup fresh cilantro, chopped

Instructions:
1. In a large pot, heat the olive oil over medium heat. Add the onion and garlic, and sauté for 3-4 minutes until softened.
2. Stir in the pumpkin puree and cook for another 5 minutes, stirring occasionally.
3. Add the cannellini beans, vegetable broth, ground cumin, and ground black pepper. Bring to a boil.
4. Reduce heat and simmer for 20-25 minutes.
5. Use an immersion blender to puree the soup until smooth.
6. Remove from heat and stir in the fresh cilantro.
7. Serve immediately.

Nutrition Info (per serving):
- Calories: 190
- Protein: 7g
- Carbohydrates: 34g
- Fat: 4g
- Fiber: 9g
- Sugar: 5g

Serves: 4
Cooking Time: 30 minutes

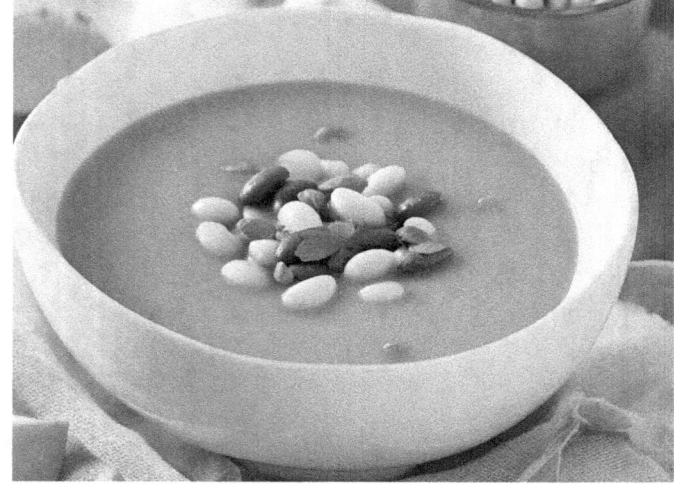

24. Chicken and Chickpea Stew

Ingredients:
- 1 tablespoon olive oil
- 1 onion, chopped
- 2 cloves garlic, minced
- 1 pound boneless, skinless chicken breast, cut into bite-sized pieces
- 1 can (15 ounces) chickpeas, rinsed and drained
- 4 cups low-sodium chicken broth
- 1 can (15 ounces) diced tomatoes (no added salt)
- 1 teaspoon ground paprika
- 1/2 teaspoon ground black pepper
- 1/4 cup fresh parsley, chopped

Instructions:
1. In a large pot, heat the olive oil over medium heat. Add the onion and garlic, and sauté for 3-4 minutes until softened.
2. Add the chicken pieces and cook until browned, about 5-7 minutes.
3. Stir in the chickpeas, chicken broth, diced tomatoes, ground paprika, and ground black pepper. Bring to a boil.
4. Reduce heat and simmer for 20-25 minutes, or until the chicken is cooked through.
5. Remove from heat and stir in the fresh parsley.
6. Serve immediately.

Nutrition Info (per serving):
- Calories: 250
- Protein: 24g
- Carbohydrates: 28g
- Fat: 6g
- Fiber: 8g
- Sugar: 6g

Serves: 4
Cooking Time: 30 minutes

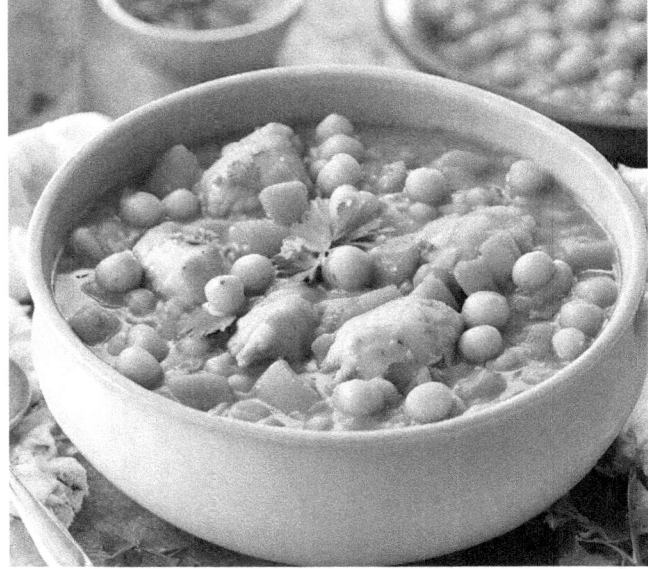

10-WEEK MEAL PLAN

Week 1
Day 1:
- Breakfast: Banana Oatmeal Smoothie
- Lunch: Chicken and Vegetable Kebabs
- Dinner: Lemon and Dill White Fish Stew

Day 2:
- Breakfast: Ginger Pear Smoothie
- Lunch: Turkey Spinach Meatloaf
- Dinner: Corn and Zucchini Chowder

Day 3:
- Breakfast: Creamy Apple-Cinnamon Smoothie
- Lunch: Grilled Chicken Caesar Salad
- Dinner: Sweet Potato and Lentil Soup

Day 4:
- Breakfast: Scrambled Egg Whites with Spinach
- Lunch: Herb Roasted Turkey Thighs
- Dinner: Broccoli and Lentil Soup

Day 5:
- Breakfast: Zucchini and Bell Pepper Frittata
- Lunch: Baked Chicken with Rosemary and Thyme
- Dinner: Kale and White Bean Soup

Day 6:
- Breakfast: Apple Sauce Pancakes
- Lunch: Chicken and Sweet Corn Soup
- Dinner: Red Lentil and Carrot Stew

Day 7:
- Breakfast: Baked Sweet Potato Hash
- Lunch: Turkey and Quinoa Stuffed Tomatoes
- Dinner: Garbanzo Bean and Vegetable Soup

Week 2
Day 8:
- Breakfast: Peach Rice Pudding
- Lunch: Chicken Piccata without Capers
- Dinner: Asparagus and White Bean Soup

Day 9:
- Breakfast: Savory Oatmeal with Poached Egg
- Lunch: Orange Rosemary Chicken
- Dinner: Pumpkin and Bean Soup

Day 10:
- Breakfast: Pumpkin Spice Oatmeal
- Lunch: Grilled Turkey Breast with Cranberry Glaze
- Dinner: Beet and Cabbage Borscht

Day 11:
- Breakfast: Herbal Tea with Rice Cakes
- Lunch: Chicken and Broccoli Alfredo
- Dinner: Turnip and Parsnip Soup

Day 12:
- Breakfast: Almond Milk Porridge
- Lunch: Chicken and Chickpea Stew
- Dinner: Mushroom and Barley Soup

Day 13:
- Breakfast: Buckwheat Pancakes
- Lunch: Steamed Chicken with Ginger and Scallions
- Dinner: Bean and Swiss Chard Stew

Day 14:
- Breakfast: Steamed Vegetable Medley
- Lunch: Balsamic Glazed Chicken Breasts
- Dinner: Fennel and Bean Stew

Week 3

Day 15:
- Breakfast: Pearled Barley Porridge
- Lunch: Chicken Soup with Barley
- Dinner: Eggplant and Tomato Stew

Day 16:
- Breakfast: Banana Rice Porridge
- Lunch: Turkey Taco Soup
- Dinner: Cauliflower and Chickpea Soup

Day 17:
- Breakfast: Egg White Omelet with Mushrooms
- Lunch: Chicken Cacciatore with Mushrooms
- Dinner: Black Bean Soup with Cilantro

Day 18:
- Breakfast: Quinoa and Berry Salad
- Lunch: Chicken and Asparagus Stir Fry
- Dinner: Watercress and Pea SouP

Day 19:
- Breakfast: Sweet Potato and Kale Smoothie
- Lunch: Grilled Chicken with Herb Marinade
- Dinner: Green Bean and Potato Soup

Day 20:
- Breakfast: Carrot and Zucchini Muffins
- Lunch: Chicken and Spinach Soup
- Dinner: Jerusalem Artichoke Soup

Day 21:
- Breakfast: Squash and Apple Bake
- Lunch: Roasted Chicken with Apples and Onions
- Dinner: Lemon Garlic Tilapia

Week 4

Day 22:
- Breakfast: Warm Barley and Pumpkin Salad
- Lunch: Grilled Chicken with Vegetable Kebabs
- Dinner: Fish Veracruz with Tomatoes and Olives

Day 23:
- Breakfast: Tapioca Pudding
- Lunch: Turkey and Quinoa Stuffed Peppers
- Dinner: Grilled Chicken with Herb Marinade

Day 24:
- Breakfast: Poached Cod with Parsley and Lemon
- Lunch: Herb Marinated Grilled Shrimp
- Dinner: Quinoa and Vegetable Soup

Day 25:
- Breakfast: Seared Scallops with Lemon Zest
- Lunch: Baked Sole with Dill
- Dinner: Chicken and Broccoli Alfredo

Day 26:
- Breakfast: Broiled Haddock with Rosemary
- Lunch: Grilled Tilapia with Herbs
- Dinner: Shrimp and Cucumber Salad

Day 27:
- Breakfast: Ginger Soy Glazed Salmon
- Lunch: Steamed Clams in White Wine
- Dinner: Roasted Chicken with Apples and Onions

Day 28:
- Breakfast: Asian Chicken Lettuce Cups
- Lunch: Turkey and Spinach Meatloaf
- Dinner: Artichoke and Potato Stew

Week 5

Day 29:
- Breakfast: Scrambled Egg Whites with Spinach
- Lunch: Turkey and Mushroom Pilaf
- Dinner: Steamed Blue Crabs

Day 30:
- Breakfast: Ginger Pear Smoothie
- Lunch: Balsamic Glazed Chicken Breasts
- Dinner: Grilled Tilapia with Herbs

Day 31:
- Breakfast: Creamy Apple-Cinnamon Smoothie
- Lunch: Turkey Spinach Meatloaf
- Dinner: Garbanzo Bean and Vegetable Soup

Day 32:
- Breakfast: Zucchini and Bell Pepper Frittata
- Lunch: Chicken Piccata without Capers
- Dinner: Lemon Garlic Tilapia

Day 33:
- Breakfast: Apple Sauce Pancakes
- Lunch: Orange Rosemary Chicken
- Dinner: Turnip and Parsnip Soup

Day 34:
- Breakfast: Baked Sweet Potato Hash
- Lunch: Grilled Chicken Caesar Salad
- Dinner: Sweet Potato and Lentil Soup

Day 35:
- Breakfast: Peach Rice Pudding
- Lunch: Chicken and Broccoli Alfredo
- Dinner: Mushroom and Barley Soup

Week 6

Day 36:
- Breakfast: Savory Oatmeal with Poached Egg
- Lunch: Turkey and Quinoa Stuffed Peppers
- Dinner: Watercress and Pea Soup

Day 37:
- Breakfast: Pumpkin Spice Oatmeal
- Lunch: Chicken and Sweet Corn Soup
- Dinner: Quinoa and Vegetable Soup

Day 38:
- Breakfast: Herbal Tea with Rice Cakes
- Lunch: Herb Marinated Grilled Shrimp
- Dinner: Black Bean Soup with Cilantro

Day 39:
- Breakfast: Almond Milk Porridge
- Lunch: Broiled Haddock with Rosemary
- Dinner: Asparagus and White Bean Soup

Day 40:
- Breakfast: Buckwheat Pancakes
- Lunch: Steamed Clams in White Wine
- Dinner: Pumpkin and Bean Soup

Day 41:
- Breakfast: Steamed Vegetable Medley
- Lunch: Shrimp and Cucumber Salad
- Dinner: Red Lentil and Carrot Stew

Day 42:
- Breakfast: Pearled Barley Porridge
- Lunch: Baked Sole with Dill
- Dinner: Eggplant and Tomato Stew

Week 7

Day 43:
- Breakfast: Banana Rice Porridge
- Lunch: Turkey and Quinoa Stuffed Tomatoes
- Dinner: Cauliflower and Chickpea Soup

Day 44:
- Breakfast: Egg White Omelet with Mushrooms
- Lunch: Chicken Cacciatore with Mushrooms
- Dinner: Beet and Cabbage Borscht

Day 45:
- Breakfast: Quinoa and Berry Salad
- Lunch: Seared Scallops with Lemon Zest
- Dinner: Green Bean and Potato Soup

Day 46:
- Breakfast: Sweet Potato and Kale Smoothie
- Lunch: Herb Roasted Turkey Thighs
- Dinner: Jerusalem Artichoke Soup

Day 47:
- Breakfast: Carrot and Zucchini Muffins
- Lunch: Grilled Chicken with Herb Marinade
- Dinner: Fennel and Bean Stew

Day 48:
- Breakfast: Squash and Apple Bake
- Lunch: Chicken and Spinach Soup
- Dinner: Lemon and Dill White Fish Stew

Day 49:
- Breakfast: Warm Barley and Pumpkin Salad
- Lunch: Baked Chicken with Rosemary and Thyme
- Dinner: Fish Veracruz with Tomatoes and Olives

Week 8

Day 50:
- Breakfast: Tapioca Pudding
- Lunch: Orange Rosemary Chicken
- Dinner: Watercress and Pea Soup

Day 51:
- Breakfast: Poached Cod with Parsley and Lemon
- Lunch: Chicken and Sweet Corn Soup
- Dinner: Broccoli and Lentil Soup

Day 52:
- Breakfast: Seared Scallops with Lemon Zest
- Lunch: Turkey Spinach Meatloaf
- Dinner: Red Lentil and Carrot Stew

Day 53:
- Breakfast: Broiled Haddock with Rosemary
- Lunch: Chicken and Asparagus Stir Fry
- Dinner: Pumpkin and Bean Soup

Day 54:
- Breakfast: Grilled Tilapia with Herbs
- Lunch: Chicken and Chickpea Stew
- Dinner: Garbanzo Bean and Vegetable Soup

Day 55:
- Breakfast: Ginger Soy Glazed Salmon
- Lunch: Steamed Clams in White Wine
- Dinner: Mushroom and Barley Soup

Day 56:
- Breakfast: Asian Chicken Lettuce Cups
- Lunch: Herb Marinated Grilled Shrimp
- Dinner: Beet and Cabbage Borscht

Week 9

Day 57:
- Breakfast: Scrambled Egg Whites with Spinach
- Lunch: Chicken Piccata without Capers
- Dinner: Green Bean and Potato Soup

Day 58:
- Breakfast: Creamy Apple-Cinnamon Smoothie
- Lunch: Chicken Soup with Barley
- Dinner: Eggplant and Tomato Stew

Day 59:
- Breakfast: Zucchini and Bell Pepper Frittata
- Lunch: Grilled Turkey Breast with Cranberry Glaze
- Dinner: Asparagus and White Bean Soup

Day 60:
- Breakfast: Apple Sauce Pancakes
- Lunch: Chicken and Vegetable Kebabs
- Dinner: Quinoa and Vegetable Soup

Day 61:
- Breakfast: Baked Sweet Potato Hash
- Lunch: Balsamic Glazed Chicken Breasts
- Dinner: Sweet Potato and Lentil Soup

Day 62:
- Breakfast: Peach Rice Pudding
- Lunch: Turkey Taco Soup
- Dinner: Turnip and Parsnip Soup

Day 63:
- Breakfast: Savory Oatmeal with Poached Egg
- Lunch: Chicken Cacciatore with Mushrooms
- Dinner: Cauliflower and Chickpea Soup

Week 10

Day 64:
- Breakfast: Pumpkin Spice Oatmeal
- Lunch: Chicken and Broccoli Alfredo
- Dinner: Fennel and Bean Stew

Day 65:
- Breakfast: Herbal Tea with Rice Cakes
- Lunch: Chicken and Spinach Soup
- Dinner: Broccoli and Lentil Soup

Day 66:
- Breakfast: Almond Milk Porridge
- Lunch: Roasted Chicken with Apples and Onions
- Dinner: Red Lentil and Carrot Stew

Day 67:
- Breakfast: Buckwheat Pancakes
- Lunch: Chicken Piccata without Capers
- Dinner: Jerusalem Artichoke Soup

Day 68:
- Breakfast: Steamed Vegetable Medley
- Lunch: Steamed Blue Crabs
- Dinner: Black Bean Soup with Cilantro

Day 69:
- Breakfast: Pearled Barley Porridge
- Lunch: Grilled Chicken Caesar Salad
- Dinner: Pumpkin and Bean Soup

Day 70:
- Breakfast: Banana Rice Porridge
- Lunch: Grilled Chicken with Herb Marinade
- Dinner: Watercress and Pea Soup

WEEKLY MEAL PLANNER + WORKBOOK

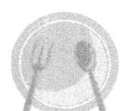

	BREAKFAST	LUNCH	DINNER	SNACKS
MONDAY				
TUESDAY				
WEDNESDAY				
THURSDAY				
FRIDAY				
SATURDAY				
SUNDAY				

What are your current dietary habits, and how do you think they might be impacting your pancreatitis?

....

....

....

....

....

....

WEEKLY MEAL PLANNER + WORKBOOK

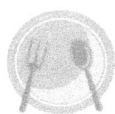

	BREAKFAST	LUNCH	DINNER	SNACKS
MONDAY				
TUESDAY				
WEDNESDAY				
THURSDAY				
FRIDAY				
SATURDAY				
SUNDAY				

What are your main goals for starting the pancreatitis-friendly diet, and what motivates you to achieve these goals?

....

....

....

....

....

....

WEEKLY MEAL PLANNER + WORKBOOK

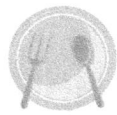

	BREAKFAST	LUNCH	DINNER	SNACKS
MONDAY				
TUESDAY				
WEDNESDAY				
THURSDAY				
FRIDAY				
SATURDAY				
SUNDAY				

List five foods you commonly eat that you will need to avoid on the pancreatitis diet. How will you feel about removing these from your diet?

....

....

....

....

....

....

WEEKLY MEAL PLANNER + WORKBOOK

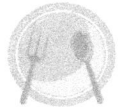

	BREAKFAST	LUNCH	DINNER	SNACKS
MONDAY				
TUESDAY				
WEDNESDAY				
THURSDAY				
FRIDAY				
SATURDAY				
SUNDAY				

Plan a week's worth of breakfasts using recipes from this cookbook. How do you feel about the variety and options available?

....

....

....

....

....

....

WEEKLY MEAL PLANNER + WORKBOOK

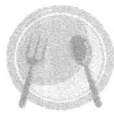

	BREAKFAST	LUNCH	DINNER	SNACKS
MONDAY				
TUESDAY				
WEDNESDAY				
THURSDAY				
FRIDAY				
SATURDAY				
SUNDAY				

Which cooking techniques or recipes in this cookbook are you most confident in preparing, and which ones seem most challenging?

....

....

....

....

....

....

WEEKLY MEAL PLANNER + WORKBOOK

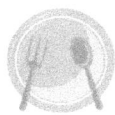

	BREAKFAST	LUNCH	DINNER	SNACKS
MONDAY				
TUESDAY				
WEDNESDAY				
THURSDAY				
FRIDAY				
SATURDAY				
SUNDAY				

Identify three flavor profiles or ingredients from the cookbook that you are most excited to try. Why do they appeal to you?

....

....

....

....

....

....

WEEKLY MEAL PLANNER + WORKBOOK

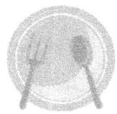

	BREAKFAST	LUNCH	DINNER	SNACKS
MONDAY				
TUESDAY				
WEDNESDAY				
THURSDAY				
FRIDAY				
SATURDAY				
SUNDAY				

How much water do you currently drink each day? What strategies can you use to ensure you stay hydrated while following this diet?

....

....

....

....

....

....

WEEKLY MEAL PLANNER + WORKBOOK

	BREAKFAST	LUNCH	DINNER	SNACKS
MONDAY				
TUESDAY				
WEDNESDAY				
THURSDAY				
FRIDAY				
SATURDAY				
SUNDAY				

How do you currently manage portion sizes, and what changes might you need to make to ensure you are eating appropriate portions?

....

....

....

....

....

....

WEEKLY MEAL PLANNER + WORKBOOK

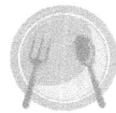

	BREAKFAST	LUNCH	DINNER	SNACKS
MONDAY				
TUESDAY				
WEDNESDAY				
THURSDAY				
FRIDAY				
SATURDAY				
SUNDAY				

What sections of the grocery store will you need to spend more time in, and which ones will you need to avoid? How will this change your shopping habits?

....

....

....

....

....

WEEKLY MEAL PLANNER + WORKBOOK

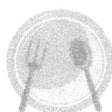

	BREAKFAST	LUNCH	DINNER	SNACKS
MONDAY				
TUESDAY				
WEDNESDAY				
THURSDAY				
FRIDAY				
SATURDAY				
SUNDAY				

What strategies can you use to stay on track with your diet when eating out at restaurants or social gatherings?

....
....
....
....
....
....

WEEKLY MEAL PLANNER + WORKBOOK

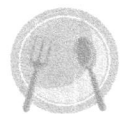

	BREAKFAST	LUNCH	DINNER	SNACKS
MONDAY				
TUESDAY				
WEDNESDAY				
THURSDAY				
FRIDAY				
SATURDAY				
SUNDAY				

Who in your life can support you in following this diet, and how can they help you stay accountable and motivated?

....

....

....

....

....

....

WEEKLY MEAL PLANNER + WORKBOOK

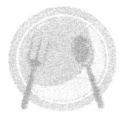

	BREAKFAST	LUNCH	DINNER	SNACKS
MONDAY				
TUESDAY				
WEDNESDAY				
THURSDAY				
FRIDAY				
SATURDAY				
SUNDAY				

Identify three potential challenges you might face while following this diet. What solutions can you think of to overcome these challenges?

....

....

....

....

....

WEEKLY MEAL PLANNER + WORKBOOK

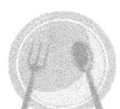

	BREAKFAST	LUNCH	DINNER	SNACKS
MONDAY				
TUESDAY				
WEDNESDAY				
THURSDAY				
FRIDAY				
SATURDAY				
SUNDAY				

After one week of following the pancreatitis diet, reflect on how you feel physically and emotionally. What positive changes have you noticed?

....

....

....

....

....

....

WEEKLY MEAL PLANNER + WORKBOOK

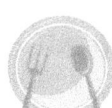

	BREAKFAST	LUNCH	DINNER	SNACKS
MONDAY				
TUESDAY				
WEDNESDAY				
THURSDAY				
FRIDAY				
SATURDAY				
SUNDAY				

How do you plan to maintain these dietary changes long-term? What strategies will you use to ensure you stick with this diet even after you have achieved your initial health goals?

....

....

....

....

....

....

Scan the QR code below to get a surprise bonus!

www.ingramcontent.com/pod-product-compliance
Lightning Source LLC
Chambersburg PA
CBHW082205220526
45470CB00010B/3049